Nanotechnology for the Regeneration of Hard and Soft Tissues

Nanotechnology for the Regeneration of Hard and Soft Tissues

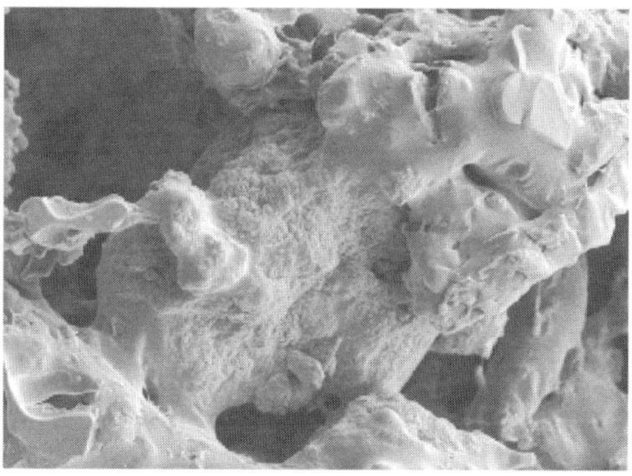

Editor

Thomas J Webster
Brown University, USA

World Scientific

NEW JERSEY • LONDON • SINGAPORE • BEIJING • SHANGHAI • HONG KONG • TAIPEI • CHENNAI

Published by

World Scientific Publishing Co. Pte. Ltd.
5 Toh Tuck Link, Singapore 596224
USA office: 27 Warren Street, Suite 401-402, Hackensack, NJ 07601
UK office: 57 Shelton Street, Covent Garden, London WC2H 9HE

British Library Cataloguing-in-Publication Data
A catalogue record for this book is available from the British Library.

NANOTECHNOLOGY FOR THE REGENERATION OF HARD AND SOFT TISSUES

ISBN-13 978-981-270-615-7
ISBN-10 981-270-615-1

Printed in Singapore by Mainland Press Pte Ltd

This book is dedicated to the next generation of learners, particularly my daughters Mia and Zoe.

Whatever the challenge, we will find solutions.

Preface

This book is centered on a topic everybody is asking. What is the commercial potential of nanotechnology? Well, look no further than the integration of nanotechnology into medicine, the so-called area of research entitled "nanomedicine". This book covers recent advances in the design, synthesis, and evaluation of nanomaterials to regenerate hard and soft tissues. Of course, when discussing how nanomaterials are being used to regenerate tissues, you cannot omit issues of toxicity. Thus, this book ends will several chapters concerning the current knowledge base of nanoparticle toxicity and how to evaluate nanoparticle toxicity.

So, then, what is the real commercial potential for nanotechnology and, in particular, nanomedicine? Depends on your definition. For example, if you think nanomedicine refers to Michael Crichton's self-replicating nanorobots traversing the body and healing disease (as in his novel *Prey* in 2002), I bet you will be waiting a long time (if ever) to see commercial fruition. On the other hand, if you envision nanomedicine referring to listening to mediation music from your nanoIPOD (and, thus, healing your soul), then your in luck as you are already experiencing commercial benefits of nanotechnology.

But if you are like the rest of us with a more reasonable interpretation of nanomedicine (the use of nanomaterials in medicine), you are somewhere in between. While it can be stated that medical fields (such as implants, imaging, diagnostics, drug delivery, etc.) are experiencing varying degrees of nanomedicine success, it is safe to say they all are beginning to see commercialization. Products have emerged. This includes various nanomaterials (nanoparticles, nanotubes, nanostructured materials, and nanocomposites), nanotools (nanolithography tools and scanning probe microscopes), and nanodevices (nanosensors and nanoelectronics) which are available commercially, and for some, human use. While to some this may not sound significant, consider for a moment the time span numerous government agencies around the world require to approve new medical devices for human use. When considering that new pharmaceuticals require up to 15 years of testing to get through the approval process (and this is just one example), it is clearly a significant advancement to even have nanomedicine products on the market.

Certainly, though, the promise of nanotechnology has created lofty expectations in some quarters. The expectations continue to grow from year to year. For example, the U.S. National Science Foundation (as one example) has contributed to this hype. The U.S. National Science Foundation is on record predicting that the market for nanotechnology, or products containing nanotechnology, will reach $1 trillion in 10 to 15 years.[1] Clearly, medical products will be a significant part of this expectation. While both advocates and opponents of nanotechnology tend to lose sight of the fact that progress in developing commercial nanotechnology applications has been understandably slow to date, the excitement is still as high (if not more) than the first day that nanomedicine emerged over ten years ago.

The expected commercial potential has not decreased or even remained the same over the past decade; it has only increased. Some have predicted that nanomedicine will exhibit strong growth in all sectors until as far out as 2011, leading to multi-billion dollar revenues.[2] Key nanomedicine technology platforms (such as nanocrystals, nanotubes, dendrimers, fullerenes, quantum dots and molecular scaffolding) are expected to drive that market expansion.[2] Few research fields have been able to sustain and grow such excitement that continues to drive nanomedicine.

So while in business and academia we are perpetually thinking of the future and asking what is real commercial potential of nanomedicine, we should not forget about where we have come. (After all, the worldwide market for nanoscale devices was 406 million dollars in 2002.[3]) Here, it is safe to say, that we have already met one important expectation: we have created products based on nanomedicine principles. Whether we will meet the continual increasing expectations of nanomedicine remains to be seen, but it is clear we have passed a significant milestone already that should put this question to rest. Such milestones and prospects for the future are emphasized in the following pages of this first-of-a-kind book. Enjoy.

References

1. http://www.biz-lib.com, accessed, January 4, 2007.

2. http://www.piribo.com, accessed, January 4, 2007.

3. http://www.bccresearch.com/editors/RB-162.html, accessed, January 4, 2007.

T. J. Webster

Contents

Preface vii

List of Contributors xix

Chapter 1 Bioinspired Nanocomposites for Orthopedic Applications 1
Huinan Liu and Thomas J. Webster

1. Introduction 1
2. Basic Science of Bone 3
   2.1. Bone Is a Nanostructured Composite 4
      2.1.1. Organic Phase: Collagen Nanofibers and Noncollagenous Proteins 4
      2.1.2. Inorganic Phase: Hydroxyapatite Nanocrystals 6
   2.2. Microstructure and Macrostructure of Bone 6
   2.3. Mechanical Properties of Bone 7
   2.4. Bone Remodeling and Bone Cells 8
      2.4.1. Osteoblasts 9
      2.4.2. Osteocytes 11
      2.4.3. Osteoclasts 11
3. Problems of Current Bone Substitutes 12
   3.1. Autografts 12
   3.2. Allografts and Xenografts 12
   3.3. Metal and Metal Alloys 12
4. Bone Tissue Engineering: Promises and Challenges 13
   4.1. Essential Requirements for Bone Scaffolds 15
      4.1.1. Biocompatibility 15

4.1.2. Biodegradability 16
4.1.3. Mechanical Properties 16
4.1.4. Surface Properties 16
4.1.5. Osteoinductivity 17
4.1.6. Interconnected Three-Dimensional Structures 17
4.1.7. Feasible Fabrication Techniques and Sterilizability 18
4.2. The Choices of Materials for Bone Scaffolds 18
4.2.1. Biodegradable Polymers 19
4.2.2. Bioactive Ceramics 25
4.2.3. Ceramic/Polymer Biocomposites 26
5. Nanocomposites: Next-Generation Materials in Orthopedics 27
5.1. Rationale and Evidence 27
5.2. Fabrication Techniques of Biocomposite Scaffolds 30
5.2.1. Solvent-Casting/Particulate-Leaching 30
5.2.2. Gas-Foaming/Particulate-Leaching 33
5.2.3. Phase Separation and Emulsion Freeze Drying 36
5.2.4. Fiber Meshes/Fiber Bonding 39
5.2.5. Melt Molding 39
5.2.6. Freeze Drying and Cross-linking 40
5.2.7. Rapid Prototyping Techniques 40
5.3. Future Directions in Orthopedics 43
Bibliography 43

Chapter 2 Nanomaterials for Better Orthopedics 53
Ganesan Balasundaram

1. Introduction 53
2. Skeletal Complications: Osteoporosis and Bone Fracture 54
3. Need for Better Implantation Materials for Orthopedic Application 55
3.1. Cell Recognition of Implant Surfaces 57
3.2. Chemistry 59
3.3. Topography 60
4. A New Approach: Nanophase Orthopedic Materials 61
4.1. Benefits of Nanophase Bone Implant Materials 66

4.2. Wettability 67
4.3. Surface Roughness 68
5. Influence of Nanomaterials Functionalized with Cell Adhesive Peptides on Osteoblast Functions 70
6. Future Challenges 72
Bibliography 74

Chapter 3 Anodization: A Promising Nano-modification Technique for Titanium for Orthopedic Applications 79
Chang Yao and Thomas J. Webster

1. Introduction 79
2. Anodization of Titanium 81
2.1. Basics of Anodization Process 81
2.2. Influences of Processing Parameters 82
2.3. Creation of Micron-Rough Surface 83
2.4. Creation of Nano-roughness 85
2.5. Control of Chemical Composition 92
3. Structure and Properties of Anodized Oxide Film 94
3.1. Structure 94
3.2. Corrosion Resistance and Adhesive Strength 96
3.3. Biological Properties of Anodized Titanium 97
3.3.1. In vitro Studies 97
3.3.2. Mechanisms of Increased Osteoblast Function 100
3.3.3. In vivo Studies 101
4. Future Directions 105
Bibliography 106

Chapter 4 Bio-inspired Carbon Nano-structures: Orthopedic Applications 111
Dongwoo Khang

1. Fundamentals of Protein Adsorption and Surface Properties 111
1.1. Adhesion Protein 113
1.2. Polar and Apolar Properties of Proteins 113
1.3. Osteoblasts 115

1.4. Carbon Nanotubes and Carbon Nanotube Composites 116
1.5. Cytocompatibility of Carbon Nanotube Composites 118
1.6. Analysis of Nano-surface Roughness 118
1.7. Role of Nano-surface Energy 119
1.8. Detecting Protein Adsorption 120
2. Protein Assisted Osteoblast Adhesion on Nanophase Materials 121
2.1. Osteoblast Functions on Carbon Nanotube Composite Materials 122
2.2. Fibronectin Attached AFM Tip Interactions on Carbon Nanotube Composite Surfaces 124
2.3. Osteoblast Functions on Micro-patterning of Carbon Nanotubes on Bio-polymers 126
3. Conclusions and Summary 130
Bibliography 130

Chapter 5 Applications of Nanotechnology/Nanomaterials in the Nervous System 135
Peishan Liu-Snyder

1. Anatomy, Physiology and Molecular Biology of the Nervous System 135
2. Epidemiology, Etiology and Pathophysiologies of Neurological Disorders 141
2.1. Spinal Cord Injury 141
2.2. Alzheimer's Disease 143
2.3. Multiple Sclerosis 146
3. Current Clinical Therapies and Limitations 147
3.1. Approved Treatments of SCI and Ongoing Human Clinical Trials 148
3.2. Pharmacological Treatments of Alzheimer's Disease and Ongoing Human Clinical Trials 149
3.3. Pharmacological Treatments of Multiple Sclerosis (MS) and Ongoing Human Clinical Trials 151
4. Application of Nanotechnology on the Development of Novel Drug and Cell Delivery Systems for the Nervous System 153

4.1. Conventional Drug Delivery Systems and Their Limitations ... 153
4.2. Advances of Nanotechnology in Drug Delivery Systems ... 154
4.3. Nano-based Matrix for Stem Cell Delivery ... 156
4.4. Medical Imaging with Nanotechnology for Early Detection and Evaluation of Treatment ... 158
5. Applications of Nanotechnologies in Electronic Tissue Interface Devices ... 161
5.1. Cochlear Implant (Bionic Ear) ... 162
5.2. Visual Prosthesis (Bionic Eye) ... 163
5.3. Computer Brain Interface (BrainGate Technology) ... 164
5.4. Functional Electrical Stimulation (FES) ... 165
5.5. Memory and Cognitive Functions ... 166
5.6. Oscillating Field Stimulator (OFS) ... 166
6. How Can Nanotechnology Improve Performance of Electronic Tissue Interface Devices? ... 167
7. Future Directions and Considerations ... 170
Bibliography ... 171

Chapter 6 Vascular Nano Stents ... 181
Karen M. Haberstroh

1. Physiology of the Vascular System ... 181
1.1. Structure and Function of the Arterial System ... 181
1.2. Components of the Artery Wall ... 182
1.3. Cells of the Vascular System ... 183
1.3.1. Vascular Endothelial Cells ... 183
1.3.2. Vascular Smooth Muscle Cells ... 184
1.3.3. Vascular Fibroblasts ... 184
1.3.4. Blood Cells ... 185
2. Atherosclerosis: A Cardiovascular Disease ... 185
2.1. The Cellular Progression of Atherosclerosis ... 186
3. Treatments for Vascular Disease ... 187
3.1. Balloon Angioplasty ... 188
3.2. Vascular Stents ... 189

3.2.1. The Use of Nano-structured Biomaterials in Vascular Stent Applications 190
3.2.2. Problems with Current Stent Designs 192
3.2.3. Stent Wear Debris 193
4. Conclusions 196
Bibliography 196

Chapter 7 Nanoparticles: Determining Toxicity 201
Ezharul Hoque Chowdhury and Toshihiro Akaike

1. Introduction 201
2. Strategies for Biocompatibility Testing 202
2.1. Cytotoxicity 202
2.2. Sensitization, Irritation and Intracutaneous Reactivity 203
2.3. Acute Systemic Toxicity 203
2.4. Genotoxicity 204
2.5. Implantation 204
2.6. Hemacompatibility 205
2.7. Subchronic and Chronic Toxicity 205
2.8. Carcinogenicity 205
2.9. Reproductive and Developmental Toxicity 206
2.10. Biodegradation 206
2.11. Immune Responses 206
3. Route of Entry and Biokinetics of Nanoparticles 207
3.1. Respiratory Tract 207
3.1.1. Alveolar Macrophage-Mediated Clearance 208
3.1.2. Translocation across Epithelial and Endothelial Cell Layers 208
3.1.3. Neural Uptake and Translocation 209
3.2. Exposure via GI Tract and Skin 210
3.3. Injection Route 210
4. Biological Adverse Effects of Nanoparticles 211
4.1. Pulmonary Effects of Nanoparticles 211
4.1.1. Pulmonary Inflammation 212
4.1.2. Pulmonary Carcinogenicity 213
4.2. Systemic Effects of Nanoparticles 214

4.3. Differences in Toxicity between Nanoparticles of Different Materials 215
4.3.1. Particle Surface Activity 216
4.3.2. Particle Agglomeration/Disagglomeration 216
5. Conclusions 216
Bibliography 217

Chapter 8 Nanoparticles: Effects on Human Health and the Environment 221
Myung-Haing Cho and Jin-Kyu Lee

1. Hopes and Concerns about Nanotechnology 221
2. Possible Adverse Health, Environment, and Safety Impacts 224
3. How to Evaluate the Toxicity of Nanoparticles? 226
4. Conclusions 231
Acknowledgements 232
Bibliography 232

Index 235

List of Contributors

Toshihiro Akaike
Professor
Department of Biomolecular Engineering
Graduate School of Bioscience and Biotechnology
Tokyo Institute of Technology
4259 Nagatsuta, Midoriku,
Yokohama 226-8501
Japan

Ganesan Balasundaram
Senior Staff Scientist
IFC Medical
2605 Fernbrook Ln N, Suite G
Plymouth, MN 55447
USA

Myung-Haing Cho
Professor
Laboratory of Toxicology
College of Veterinary Medicine
Nano Systems Institute–National Core Research Center
Seoul National University
Seoul 151-742
Korea

Ezharul Hoque Chowdhury
PhD Candidate
Department of Biomolecular Engineering
Graduate School of Bioscience and Biotechnology
Tokyo Institute of Technology
4259 Nagatsuta, Midoriku,
Yokohama 226-8501
Japan

Karen M. Haberstroh
Director of STEM Outreach and Assistant Professor
Division of Engineering
Brown University
184 Hope Street
Providence, RI 02917
USA

Dongwoo Khang
Post-Doctoral Researcher
Division of Engineering
Brown University
184 Hope Street
Providence, RI 02917
USA

Jin-Kyu Lee
Professor
Materials Chemistry Laboratory
School of Chemistry
Nano Systems Institute–National Core Research Center
Seoul National University
Seoul 151-742
Korea

Huinan Liu
PhD Candidate
Division of Engineering
Brown University
184 Hope Street
Providence, RI 02917
USA

Peishan Liu-Snyder
Post-Doctoral Researcher
Division of Engineering
Brown University
184 Hope Street
Providence, RI 02917
USA

Thomas J. Webster
Associate Professor
Division of Engineering and Department of Orthopedic Surgery
Brown University
184 Hope Street
Providence, RI 02917
USA

Chang Yao
PhD Candidate
Division of Engineering
Brown University
184 Hope Street
Providence, RI 02917
USA

Chapter 1

Bioinspired Nanocomposites for Orthopedic Applications

Huinan Liu and Thomas J. Webster

1. Introduction

An estimated 1.5 million individuals in the United States suffer a fracture caused by some form of bone disease annually.[1] Most adverse effects of bone diseases relate to fractures. Osteoporosis is a leading underlying cause of bone fractures which affect both males and females at all ages, although to varying degrees. Other bone disorders, such as Paget's disease, osteogenesis imperfecta, rickets, and osteomalacia also have adverse influences on bone structure, strength, and density, and subsequently lead to bone fractures.

Orthopedic prostheses are often required to repair or replace damaged bone tissue due to those diseases, injuries or genetic malformations. In 2001, about 165,000 hip joints and 326,000 knees were replaced in hospitals in the United States according to the National Center for Health Statistics.[2] Direct care expenditures for fractures such as surgery and therapy cost approximately 18 billion dollars per year in the United States. Indirect costs such as lost productivity for patients may add billions of dollars to this figure.[1] In the coming decades, these costs could increase in double or triple if surgical removal and revisions become necessary after implantation when an orthopedic implant fails under physiological loading conditions. A majority of those patients who receive an orthopedic implant may have to undergo several revision surgeries in their lifetime since the average longevity of current orthopedic implants is only 10 to 15 years.[3] Therefore, in order to decrease patient discomfort and costs, designing the next generation of orthopedic prostheses with improved clinical efficacy and longer effective lifetimes is a principal task of researchers in the biomaterials field.

Over the past 25 years, researchers have been interested in applying composites to satisfy a wide diversity of biomedical demands considering that living tissue are composed of composites with a number of levels of hierarchy. In almost all biological systems a range of properties is required, such as physicochemical properties, mechanical properties, and biological activity, which are all of great importance to the clinical success of biomaterials. The development of bioinspired nanocomposites offers the great promise to improve the efficacy of current orthopedic implants. Specifically, for organic/inorganic biocomposites, it is possible to obtain a wide range of mechanical and biological properties by modifying the type and distribution of inorganic phase in the organic matrix and hence to optimize the performance of the biomedical devices and their interaction with the host tissues. A wide variety of biocomposites have been synthesized and fabricated for various biomedical applications during these years. The general class of organic/inorganic nanocomposites is a fast growing area of research. Significant effort is focused on the ability to obtain control of the nano-scale structures via innovative synthetic approaches. The properties of nano-composite materials depend not only on the properties of their individual components but also on their fabrication techniques which have significant influences on the structure, morphology, distribution of phases and interfacial characteristics of nanocomposites.

For potential applications to be successful, full advantage must be taken of the comprehensive properties of biocomposites and the advanced manufacturing techniques to meet the needs of biomedical applications. This chapter systematically addresses nanocomposites applied to repair or replace damaged bone tissue in a comprehensive manner, and emphasizes on the influence of nanotechnology on fabrication of nanocomposites and their applications in tissue engineering.

This chapter focuses on three main areas. First, it introduces natural bone and widely used synthetic composites in natural bone repair. Second, the requirements of biocomposites in nano-scale structures for tissue engineering applications are described. The third area concerns manufacturing techniques of various bioinspired nanocomposites, including examples of the design and fabrication of three-dimensional composite scaffolds for tissue engineering applications.

2. Basic Science of Bone

One approach to develop better orthopedic materials is to mimic or closely match the composition, microstructure and properties of natural bone. Bone has a varied arrangement of material structures at different length scales which work in concert to perform diverse mechanical, biological and chemical functions; such as structural support, protection and storage of healing cells, and mineral ion homeostasis.

Scale is very important in describing hierarchical architecture of bone and understanding relationship between structures at various levels of hierarchy. There are 3 levels of structures: (1) the nanostructure (a few nanometers to a few hundred nanometers), such as non-collagenous organic proteins, fibrillar collagen and embedded mineral crystals; (2) the microstructure (from 1 to 500 micrometers), such as lamellae, osteons, and Haversian systems; (3) the macrostructure, such as cancellous and cortical bone. These three levels of oriented structures assemble into the heterogeneous and anisotropic bone, as shown in Fig. 1.

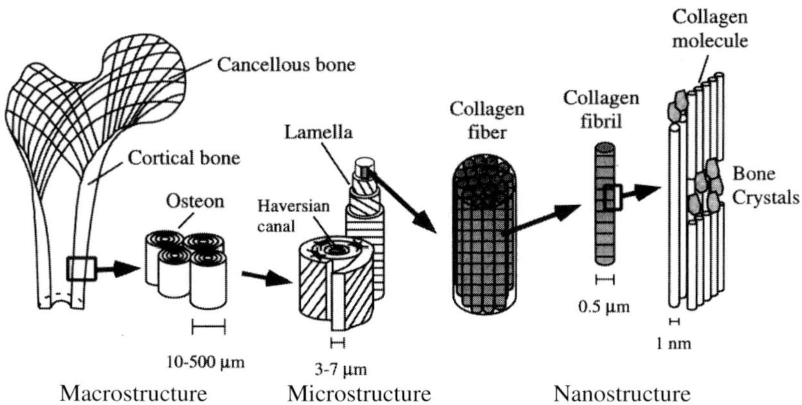

Figure 1. Schematic structure of a human femur. (Adapted and redrawn from[4]).

In this manner, it is important to first understand the nanostructured components of bone.

2.1. Bone Is a Nanostructured Composite

Natural bone is a composite material composed of organic compounds (mainly collagen) reinforced with inorganic compounds (minerals). The most prominent structures seen at nano-scale are the collagen fibers, surrounded and infiltrated by minerals. Bone builds its hierarchical architecture from these nanostructured building blocks. The detailed composition of bone differs depending on species, age, dietary history, health status and anatomical location. In general, however, the inorganic phase accounts for about 70% of the dry weight of bone and the organic matrix makes up the remainder.[5]

2.1.1. Organic Phase: Collagen Nanofibers and Noncollagenous Proteins

Approximately 90% of the organic phase of bone is Type I collagen; the remaining 10% consists of noncollagenous proteins and ground substances.

Type I Collagen found in bone is synthesized by osteoblasts (bone-forming cells) and is secreted as a triple helical procollagen into the extracellular matrix, where collagen molecules are stabilized by cross-linking of reactive aldehydes among the collagen chains. Generally, each of the 12 types of collagen found in body consists of 3 polypeptide chains composed of approximately 1,000 amino acids each. Specifically, Type I collagen (molecular weight 139,000 Daltons) possesses 2 identical $\alpha 1(I)$ chains and 1 unique $\alpha 2$ chain; this configuration produces a fairly rigid linear molecule that is 300 nm long.[6] The linear molecules (or fibers) of Type I collagen are self-assembled in triple helix bundles having a periodicity of 67 nm, with 40 nm gaps (called hole-zones) between the ends of the molecules and pores between the sides of parallel molecules, as shown in Fig. 2. The collagen fibers provide the framework and architecture of bone while the hydroxyapatite (HA) crystals located in the fibers and between the fibers.

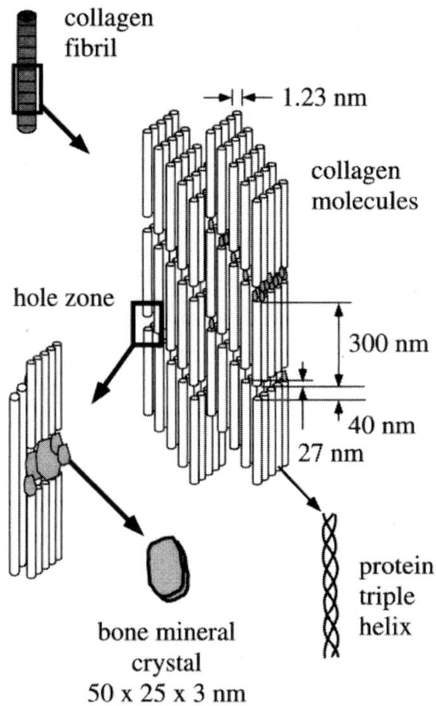

Figure 2. A schematic diagram illustrating the assembly of collagen fibers and bone mineral crystals. (Adapted and redrawn from[4]).

Noncollagenous proteins, for example, growth factors and cytokines (such as insulin-like growth factors and osteogenic proteins), bone inductive proteins (such as osteonectin, osteopontin, and osteocalcin), and extracellular matrix compounds (such as bone sialoprotein, bone proteoglycans, and other phosphoproteins as well as proteolipids) provide minor contributions to the overall weight of bone but have majorcontributions to its biological functions, such as regulate the size and orientation of the minerals, serve as a reservoir for calcium and phosphate ions, etc. During new bone formation, noncollagenous proteins are synthesized by osteoblasts and mineral ions (such as calcium and phosphate) are deposited into the hole-zones and pores of the collagen matrix to promote HA crystal growth. The ground substance is formed from proteins, polysaccharides and mucopolysaccharides which acts as a cement, filling the spaces between collagen fibers and HA crystals.

2.1.2. Inorganic Phase: Hydroxyapatite Nanocrystals

The inorganic or mineral component of bone is primarily crystalline hydroxyapatite, $Ca_{10}(PO_4)_6(OH)_2$ or HA. Plate-like HA nanocrystals of bone locate at the discrete spaces (hole zones) within the collagen fibrils, thereby limiting the possible primary growth of the mineral crystals, and forcing the crystals to be discrete and discontinuous. The mineral crystals grow with a specific crystalline orientation, that is, the c axes of the crystals are roughly parallel to the long axes of the collagen fibrils.[7] The average lengths and widths of the plates are 50 x 25 nm. Crystal thickness is 2-3 nm.[4]

Small amounts of impurities which affect cellular functions may be present in the mineralized HA matrix; for example, magnesium, strontium, sodium, or potassium ions may replace calcium ions, carbonate may replace phosphate groups, whereas chloride and fluoride may replace hydroxyl groups. Because the release of ions from the mineral bone matrix controls cell-mediated functions, the presence of impurities may alter certain physical properties of bone such as solubility and consequently important biological aspects which are critical to normal bone function. For example, magnesium present in the mineralized matrix may enhance cellular activity and promote growth of HA crystals and subsequent new bone formation.[1]

In conclusion, bone itself is a nanostructured composite composed of nanometer sized HA well-dispersed in a mostly collagen matrix (Fig. 2). Although the inorganic and organic components of bone have structural and some regulatory functions, the principal regulators of bone metabolism are bone cells which will be discussed in section 2.4.

2.2. Microstructure and Macrostructure of Bone

At the microstructural level, bone consists of two structures: woven and lamellae. Woven bone is immature or a primitive form of bone and is normally found in the metaphyseal region of growing bone as well as in fracture callus and diseased (such as Pagetic) bone. Woven bone is composed of relatively disoriented coarse collagen fibers and thus has isotropic characteristics. In contrast, lamellae bone is a more mature bone that results from the remodeling of woven or previously existing bone. Bone lamellae with approximate 3-7 μm in thickness is highly organized and contains stress-oriented collagen fibers which lies in parallel in each lamella and results in anisotropic properties with greatest strength parallel to the longitudinal axis of the collagen fibers. These collagen fibers change the orientation from one lamella to another, which is described figuratively as a twisted plywood or helicoidal structure.[8] Lamellae bone is formed into concentric rings (approximately 4-20 rings) called osteons with a central blood supply called a Haversian system.

At the macrostructure level, bone is distinguished into the cortical (or compact) and cancellous (or spongy) types. In cross-section, the end of a long bone such as the femur has a dense cortical shell with a porous, cancellous interior.[9] Flat bones such as the calvaria have a sandwich structure: dense cortical layers on the outer surfaces and a thin, reinforcing cancellous structure within. Cancellous bone is characterized by a three-dimensional sponge-like branching lattice structure with 50 to 90% porosity and large pores which are up to several millimeters in diameter. Cancellous bone, primarily found at the epiphyses and metaphyses of both long and cuboidal bones, approximates an isotropic material and mainly receives compression under physiological loading conditions. In contrast, cortical bone is characterized by less than 30% porosity and is composed of small pores up to 1 mm in diameter. Compact bone, primarily found at the diaphysis of long bones such as the femur and the tibia, is highly anisotropic with reinforcing structures along its loading axis. In general, cancellous bone is much more active metabolically, is remodeled more often than cortical bone, and is therefore "younger" on average than cortical bone.

2.3. Mechanical Properties of Bone

Cortical bone is usually more dense and, thus, mechanically stronger than cancellous bone. The relative density and some mechanical

Table 1. Relative density and mechanical properties of healthy human bone. (Adapted and redrawn from[10-12]).

	Cancellous Bone	Cortical Bone (Longitude)	Cortical Bone (Transverse)
Relative Density	0.05-0.7	0.7-1.8	
Elongation (%)	5-7	1-3	
Elastic Modulus (GPa)	0.1-0.5	17-30	7-13
Ultimate Tensile Strength (MPa)	2-20	130-150	50-60

properties of bone are shown in Table 1. These properties also change with sex, age, dietary history, health status, and anatomical locations. The anisotropic ratio for whole bone is usually between 2.1 and 2.6 in longitudinal and transversal directions.[10] Diseased bone usually has lower density and weaker mechanical properties than respective healthy bone.

2.4. Bone Remodeling and Bone Cells

It is not only the complex architecture of natural bone that makes it difficult to replace, but also its dynamic ability. Bone has the ability regenerate when damaged and also to remodel when the loading conditions change, for example, the mass of bone mineral can be increased with exercise, making bones less likely to fracture.[13] Therefore, it is important to understand how bone cells coordinate during this bone remodeling process.

Bone as a living organ can change in size, shape, position, and properties by its remodeling process throughout their lifetimes to respond to different kinds of stress produced by physical activity or mechanical loads. Therefore, bone has the capability of self-repairing under excessive mechanical stresses by activating the remodeling process through the formation of a bone-modeling unit (BMU). This process involves three major types of bone cells: osteoblasts (bone-forming cells), osteocytes (bone-maintaining cells), and osteoclasts (bone-resorbing cells).

Figure 3 depicts how bone cells cooperate in the bone remodeling process.[14] Osteoclasts are activated by growth factors, cytokines, and proteins present in the bone matrix to resorb old bone. Osteoblasts are then activated by growth factors such as insulin-like growth factors I and II secreted by osteoclasts and/or osteocytes to deposit calcium-containing minerals. Osteocytes regulate new bone formation by modulating osteoblast differentiation from non-calcium depositing to calcium depositing cells through secretion of growth factors such as insulin-like growth factor I and the tissue growth factor β.[15]

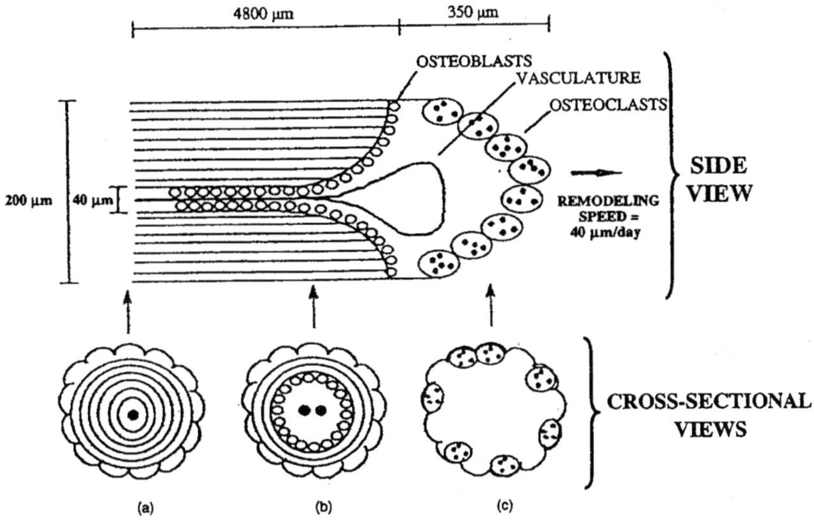

Figure 3. Schematic diagram of coordinated bone cell functions that maintain homeostasis during bone remodeling. (Adapted and redrawn from[14]).

2.4.1. Osteoblasts

Osteoblasts are located on the periosteal and endosteal surfaces of bone with an average diameter of 10 to 50 μm and contribute to new bone synthesis. Fig. 4 schematically describes the time course of osteoblast proliferation and differentiation on a newly implanted biomaterial. After initial adhesion to the surface of an implant, osteoblasts actively proliferate and express genes for Type I collagen, vitronectin, and fibronectin. At the end of proliferation, the extracellular matrix development and maturation begin and osteoblasts start to differentiate from non-calcium to calcium depositing cells. Alkaline phosphatase activity and mRNA expression for proteins (such as osteopontin, and collagenase) are increased tenfold. As the mineralization process begins and mineral nodules form, osteoblasts synthesize and deposit bone sialoprotein, osteocalcin (a calcium-binding protein), and other matrix proteins. Osteocalcin interacts with HA and is thought to mediate coupling to bone resorption by osteoclasts and bone formation by osteoblasts and/or osteocytes.

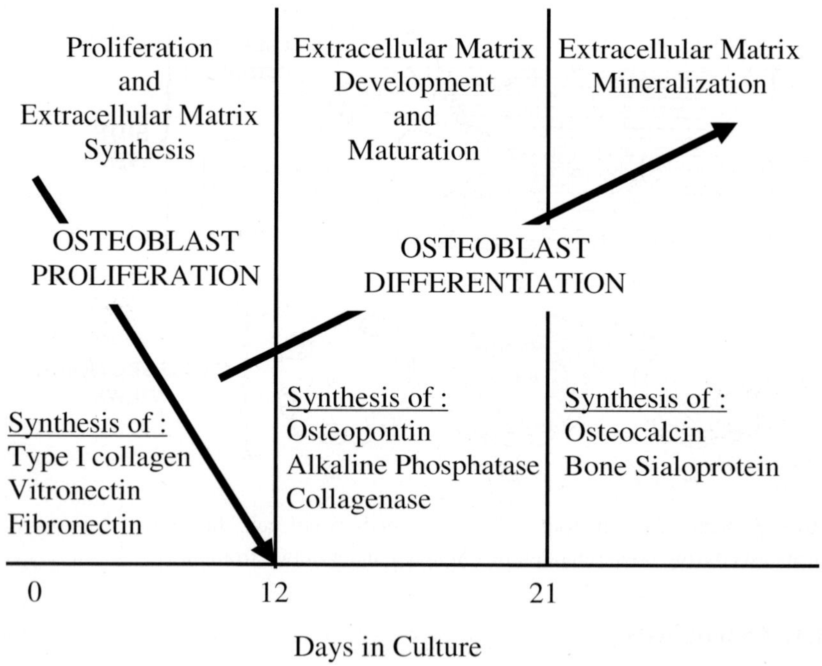

Figure 4. Time course of osteoblast functions on a newly implanted biomaterial. (Adapted and redrawn from[16]).

2.4.2. Osteocytes

Osteocytes are mature osteoblasts embedded in mineralized bone matrix and also contribute to new bone synthesis but to a lesser extent than osteoblasts. The principal difference between osteocytes and osteoblasts is their relative location in bone. Osteocytes are arranged concentrically around the central lumen of an osteon and in between lamellae (Fig. 1). Osteocytes possess extensive long branches with which they establish contacts and communications with adjacent osteocytes through small channels called canaliculi. Due to their three-dimensional distribution and interconnecting structure, osteocytes are believed to be sensitive to physiological stress and strain signals in bone tissue and help to mediate or balance (i) osteoblastic activity to deposit new bone and (ii) osteoclastic activity to dissolve old bone.

2.4.3. Osteoclasts

Osteoclasts are derived from pluripotent cells of bone marrow and lie in the regions of bone resorption in pits called Howship's lacunae. Osteoclasts, primarily responsible for bone resorption, are distinguished by their large size which is up to 100 μm in diameter and their multiple nuclei which could be up to 100 per cell. When osteoclasts sweep across disrupted bone surfaces to dissolve bone, they first form ruffled cell membrane edges to increases their total surface area of attachment onto the resorptive surfaces. Then, osteoclasts produce tartrate-resistant acid phosphatase (also know as TRAP) which results in the release of hydrogen ions through the carbonic anhydrase system and subsequently decreases the pH of the local environment. The lowered pH increases the solubility of HA crystals and the organic component of bone matrix are removed lastly by acidic proteolytic digestion.

Importantly, the extent of bone remodeling that occurs at an implant surface will determine the fate of the prosthetic device. For example, loosening and failure of the implant may result from either: (1) little or no remodeling in the bone surrounding an implant, which may lead to malnourished juxtaposed bone, or (2) too much remodeling in the bone surrounding an implant, which may lead to excessive bone resorption, or osteolysis.

3. Problems of Current Bone Substitutes

Traditionally, autografts, allografts, xenografts and metal implants have been used to repair fractures and other bone defects. However, these substitutes are far from ideal as each has its own specific problems and limitations.[17]

3.1. Autografts

Autograft is the tissue removed from one portion of the skeleton and transferred to another location in the same individual. It is commonly taken in the form of cancellous bone from the patient's iliac crest, but compact bone can be used as well.[18] Historically, autografts have been the gold standard of bone replacement for many years because they provide osteogenic cells as well as essential osteoinductive factors needed for bone healing and regeneration. However, autografts are always associated with donor shortage and donor site morbidity, which severely limit its applications. The number of patients requiring a transplant far exceeds the available supply of donor tissue.[19] New technology is needed to reduce this deficit.

3.2. Allografts and Xenografts

Allograft is the tissue transplanted between genetically non-identical members of the same species while a xenograft is the tissue transplanted between members of different species. Clearly, allografts and xenografts have the risk of disease transmission and immune response.[20,21]

3.3. Metal and Metal Alloys

Due to the above stated issues with autografts, allografts, and xenografts, synthetic materials such as metals have been the material of choice for numerous orthopedic applications for a long time. However, metal and metal alloys can not perform as well as healthy bone and can not remodel or self-repair with time because they do not exhibit the physiological, dynamic and mechanical characteristics of true bone.

Table 2 highlights some physical and mechanical properties of metals which are currently used for orthopedic implants. Obviously, metals have much higher density and mechanical properties than true bone previously listed in Table 1.

Table 2. Selected physical and mechanical properties of metal alloys. (Adapted and redrawn from[22]).

	Stainless Steel (316L Annealed)	CoCrMo(F75 Cast)	Ti6Al4V
Density (g/cm^3)	8	8.3	4.42
Elastic Modulus (GPa)	193	220	100
Yield Strength (MPa)	172	450	795
Ultimate Tensile Strength (MPa)	485	655	860
Elongation (%)	40	8	10

Mismatches in the mechanical properties of metallic implants and physiological bone result in "stress shielding" problems.[23] That is, the implanted material shields the healing bone from mechanical loading, resulting in necrosis of the surrounding bone and subsequent implant loosening. This condition creates clinical complications and necessitates additional surgery to remove implants and necrotic bone tissue. In addition to the "stress shielding" problems, insufficient osseointegration or lack of strongly bonded bone to the material surface may also lead to either loosening of implants or ingrowth of fibrous tissue. Both outcomes may consequently lead to clinical failure and further revision surgery.

All these clinical problems that are major obstacles to overcome emphasize a critical need for novel synthetic bone substitutes with similar structure, properties, and functions as physiological bone.

4. Bone Tissue Engineering: Promises and Challenges

Bone tissue engineering, which typically involves the assembly of bone structures by combining bone cells and scaffolds, offers a promising opportunity for bone regeneration in a natural way. Tissue engineering is a new evolving discipline that has been described as: "the application of principles of engineering and life sciences towards a fundamental understanding of structure-function relationships in normal and pathological mammalian tissues and the development of biological substitutes to restore, maintain, or improve tissue function".[24] In tissue engineering, tissue substitutes are constructed in the laboratory by combining living cells with artificial components such as biomaterials which are subsequently introduced into a patient to create, repair or replace natural tissues and/or organs. Fig. 5 shows the bone tissue engineering concept using a hypothetical example of a femur.[25] Ideal scaffolds should be biodegradable and are designed as a temporary 3D mirror matrix, onto which cells grow and regenerate the needed tissues. The scaffolds will resorb after fulfilling the template functions and thus nothing foreign will be left in these patients.

Currently, the scientific challenges of bone tissue engineering are: (i) developing suitable 3D scaffolds that act as templates for cell adhesion, growth and proliferation in favored 3D orientations and (ii) understanding cell functions on these scaffolds.[26] The scaffolds provide the necessary support for the cells to proliferate and differentiate, and their architectures define the ultimate shapes of new bones. Over the past decade, one of the main goals of bone tissue engineering has been to develop biodegradable materials as bone substitutes for filling large bone defects. In addition, such scaffolds must allow for proper diffusion of oxygen and nutrients to cells embedded into the scaffold as well as proper diffusion of waste from the cells. The final goal is to return full biological and mechanical functionality to a damaged bone tissue.

Scaffolds, as essential components for tissue engineering strategies, must have a series of suitable properties for bone regeneration purposes. Successful design of scaffolds involves comprehensive consideration of macro and micro-structural properties of the scaffolds and their interactions with natural tissue at nano-scale range. Such properties affect not only cell survival, proliferation, signaling, growth, and differentiation but also their gene expression and the preservation of their phenotype, which eventually determines clinical healing success or failure.

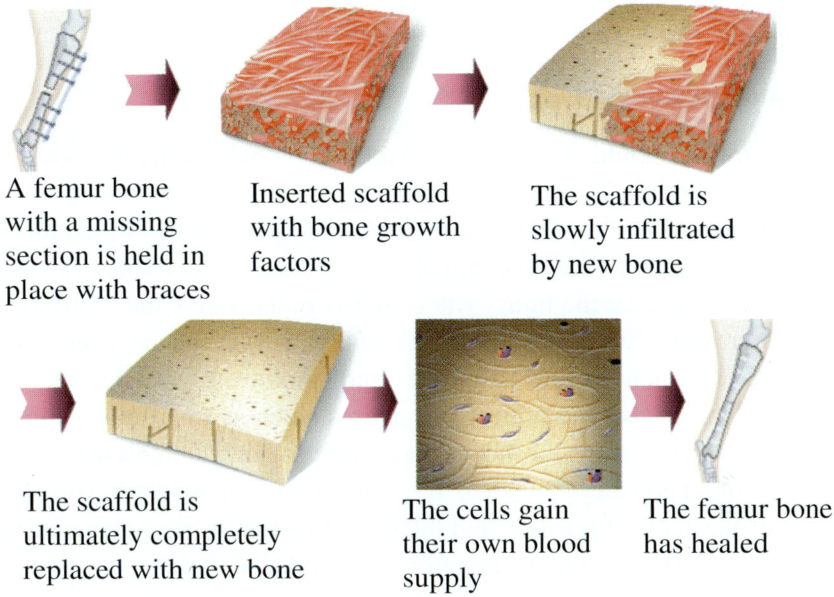

Figure 5. Schematic diagram of bone tissue engineering concept. (Adapted and redrawn from[25]).

4.1. Essential Requirements for Bone Scaffolds

When developing a scaffold for use in orthopedics, the properties highlighted in the following sections are critical considerations.

4.1.1. Biocompatibility

The scaffolds should be biocompatible to the cells and be well integrated into the host tissue without eliciting an immune response, cytotoxicity, or formation of scar tissue. [18] Factors that determine biocompatibility can be affected by scaffold or polymer synthesis and fabrication techniques. For example, residual chemicals involved in polymer processes (such as organic solvents, initiators, stabilizers, cross-linking agents, or unreacted monomers) may leach out of the scaffold once implanted. Therefore, not only the intact biomaterial, but also any leachable components and degradation products, must be biocompatible. Specifically, the release of acidic by-products from some scaffold materials, cause tissue necrosis or inflammation due to a quick drop in local pH.[27]

4.1.2. Biodegradability

The scaffolds should be biodegradable and bioresorbable with a controllable degradation and resorption rate to match cell/tissue growth *in vitro* and *in vivo*. The degradation rate of the scaffolds and the rate of new tissue formation must be coupled appropriately to each other in such a way that by the time the injury site is totally regenerated, the scaffold is totally degraded. The degradation rate of a scaffold can be altered by many factors such as its structure and molecular weight of the component materials. The scaffold structures (such as surface-to-volume ratio, porosity, pore size and shape) play a role in degradation kinetics, as does scaffold geometry. *In vivo*, the choice of implantation site, the amount of mechanical loading, and the rate of metabolism of degradation products also influence the degradation time of the scaffolds.

4.1.3. Mechanical Properties

The scaffolds should have adequate mechanical properties to match the intended site of implantation. *In vitro*, the scaffolds should have sufficient mechanical strength to withstand hydrostatic pressures and to maintain spacing required for cell in-growth and matrix production.[28] *In vivo*, because bone is always under physiological stresses (such as compression, tension, torsion, and bending), the mechanical properties of the implanted scaffolds should closely match those of living bone so that an early healing of the injured site can be made possible.

4.1.4. Surface Properties

The scaffolds should have appropriate surfaces to favor cell attachment, proliferation and differentiation. Surface properties, both chemical and topographical, can control and affect bioactivity and osteoconductivity. Chemical properties are related to the ability of proteins to initially adsorb and subsequently for cells to adhere to the material surface. Topographical properties are of particular interest when osteoconductivity is concerned. Osteoconduction is the process by which osteogenic cells migrate to the surface of the scaffold through a fibrin clot, which is established right after the material implantation. This migration of osteogenic cells through the clot will cause retraction of the temporary fibrin matrix. Hence, it is of the utmost importance that the fibrin matrix is well secured to the scaffolds, otherwise, when osteogenic cells start to migrate, the fibrin will detach from the scaffolds due to wound contraction. As opposed to a smooth surface it has been previously shown that a more ''rough'' surface will be able to imprison the fibrin matrix and hence facilitate the migration of osteogenic cells to the scaffold surface.[29,30]

4.1.5. Osteoinductivity

Osteoinduction is the process by which mesenchymal stem and pluripotent osteoprogenitor cells are recruited to a bone healing site. It is the hope that they are then stimulated to the osteogenic differentiation pathway. However, when the portion of bone that requires regeneration is large, natural osteoinduction combined with a biodegradable scaffold may be not enough. Therefore, the scaffold itself should be osteoinductive to promote bone formation. Recombinant human bone morphogenetic proteins (rhBMPs), such as rhBMP-2 and rhBMP-7, were found osteoinductive and capable of inducing new bone formation. Recent researches demonstrated that combining rhBMPs with the scaffolds could significantly increase osteoinductivity of the scaffolds and hence promote new bone growth.[31]

4.1.6. Interconnected Three-Dimensional Structures

The scaffolds should be three-dimensional and highly porous with appropriate scaled interconnected pores to favor vascularization, tissue integration, and flow transport of nutrients and metabolic waste. Pore size is a very important property because the scaffolds with large void volume and large surface-area-to-volume ratio maximize space to help cells, tissues, and blood vessels penetrate. To attain a high surface area per unit volume, however, smaller pores are preferable as long as the pore size is greater than the diameter of osteoblasts (typically 10 μm). If the pores employed are too small, pore occlusion by the cells may happen. This will prevent cellular penetration and neovascularization of the inner areas of the scaffold. It is reported that interconnected larger pores facilitate diffusion and cell migration within the scaffolds, improving nutrient supply and waste removal, and thus increasing the viability of cells at the center of the scaffolds. [27] Currently, researchers are still searching for optimal pore size and shape for various tissue engineering applications. It is also crucial to control the suitable porosity of scaffolds by adjusting available fabrication techniques to match the porosity of true bone. Importantly, the porosity, pore structures, and pore size affect the mechanical and biological properties of scaffolds.

4.1.7. Feasible Fabrication Techniques and Sterilizability

The scaffolds should be fabricated reproducibly on a large scale from versatile processing techniques for a variety of shapes and sizes to match bone defects in the patients. As with all implanted materials, the scaffolds must be easily sterilizable to prevent infection. The method of sterilization, however, must not interfere with bioactivity of biomaterials or alter their chemical composition, which could influence their biocompatibility or degradation properties.

Bearing these requirements in mind, several popular materials for bone tissue engineering applications will be further discussed in the next section.

4.2. The Choices of Materials for Bone Scaffolds

The selection of the most appropriate material to produce a scaffold to be used in bone tissue engineering applications is a very important step towards the construction of a successful tissue-engineered product. As mentioned, the properties of constituent materials will determine, to a great extent, the properties of the scaffolds. So far, a wide variety of natural and synthetic biomaterials, such as polymers, ceramics, and a combination of them, have been studied for bone tissue engineering applications. Table 3 highlights some physical and mechanical properties of materials of particular interest for bone repair.

Table 3. Material properties. (Redrawn from[32-35].)

Materials	Density (g/cm^3)	Elastic Modulus (GPa)	Ultimate Strength (MPa)
Polymers			
Polyethylene (PE)	0.91-0.96	0.88-1	30-35 (Tensile)
Poly(methyl methacrylate) (PMMA)	1.15-1.2	2.1-3.4	22-48 (Tensile) 64-103 (Compressive)
Tyrosine-derived Polycarbonate	1.2	1.2-1.5	51-67 (Tensile)
Ceramics			
Alumina	3.8-4.0	365-380	6-55 (Tensile) 1000-2700 (Compressive)
Zirconia	5.7-5.95	190-210	>300 (Tensile) 1500-2000 (Compressive)
HA	3.15-3.22	40-117	8-50 (Tensile) 100-294 (Compressive)
Composites			
Epoxy/carbon fiber	1.55-1.63	46-215	579-1240 (Tensile)
Polypropylene fumarate/ Tricalcium phosphate (PPF/TCP)	N/A	0.4-1.2	16.7-17.9 (Compressive)
Bioglass®	2.2-3.7	35	42-84 (Tensile)

4.2.1. Biodegradable Polymers

Bioresorbable natural and synthetic polymers have attracted increasing attention for their use as scaffold materials in the last ten years.[36] Many practical advantages arise because these polymers such as PLGA (poly-lactide-co-glycolide) allow for precise control of chemical composition (e.g., the lactide/glycolide ratio in the PLGA copolymers), crystallinity, molecular weight, molecular weight distribution, as well as microstructure and macrostructure (including porosity).[37-39] This allows adequate control of scaffold properties (such as degradation rate and mechanical strength), thus creating optimal conditions for cell survival, proliferation, and subsequent tissue formation. The degradation products of these polymers can be removed by natural metabolic pathways.

The most commonly used synthetic polymers are biodegradable aliphatic polyesters. Poly(glycolic acid) (PGA, also called as polyglycolide), poly(lactic acid) (PLA, also called as polylactide), and their copolymers poly(lactic-co-glycolic acid) (PLGA, also called as poly-lactide-co-glycolide), as a family of aliphatic polyesters, are some of the most popular scaffold polymers.[40-42]

PLGA was originally developed for use in resorbable surgical sutures and biodegradable drug delivery systems. These polymers (PLA, PGA, and PLGAs) are approved by the U.S. Food and Drug Administration (FDA) for certain human clinical applications. The first commercial suture, Dexon® (composed of poly-lactide-co-glycolide), was available in 1970 and the first FDA-cleared drug product was the Lupron Depot drug-delivery system (TAP Pharmaceutical Products Inc.; Lake Forest, IL) which was a controlled release device for the treatment of advanced prostate cancer that used biodegradable microspheres of 75/25 lactide/glycolide to administer leuprolide acetate over periods of time up to 4 months (replacing daily injections). Since then there has been intensive development of medical devices composed of PGA, PLA, and their copolymers.[43] The use of biodegradable polymers in orthopedic devices for fixation of fractures of long bones was first clinically implemented in Finland in 1984.[44,45] Since the 1990s, the applications of PLA, PGA, and PLGAs in tissue engineering have been investigated extensively.[46]

DL-Lactides and glycolides are polymerized via a cationic ring-opening reaction in the presence of stannous octoate as a catalyst to form a random copolymer called poly(DL-lactide-co-glycolide) or PLGA. A representative polymerization reaction is shown in Fig. 6. PLGA gradually degrades into the endogenous natural metabolites lactic acid and glycolic acid by non-enzymatic hydrolysis of ester bonds in its backbone.[47,48] The polymers that undergo hydrolytic cleavage tend to have more predictable degradation rates *in vivo* than polymers whose degradation is mediated predominantly by enzymes because the levels of enzymatic activity may vary widely not only among different patients but also among different tissue sites in the same patient. But, the availability of water is virtually constant in all soft/hard tissues and varies little from patient to patient. The degradation products of PGA, PLA and PLGA are nontoxic, natural metabolites, and are eventually eliminated from the body in the form of carbon dioxide and water.

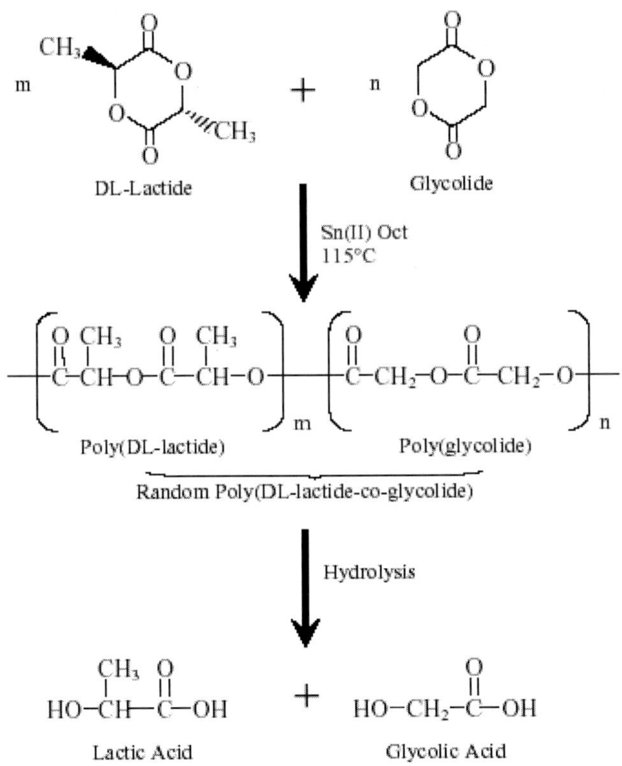

Figure 6. Synthesis of poly(DL-lactide-co-glycolide) (PLGA) and decomposition into respective acids by hydrolysis.

The PLGA degradation process has been divided into four steps that begins at the outer perimeter of the device and moves gradually into the interior, followed by catastrophic disintegration.[49] In step 1, water diffuses into the polymer and hydrolytic random chain scission of ester bonds start. In step 2, differentiation between the surface and interior begins, with a drastic decrease in molecular weight in the inner part of the matrix, where the acidic environment accelerates the degradation. In step 3, low-molecular-weight oligomers begin to diffuse through the thinning outer layer, and when the molecular weight of these oligomers is low enough to allow the solubilization in the medium, weight loss begins. In the final step 4, a polymer shell remains after the oligomers have solubilized and slow degradation of the shell takes place. Degradation of PLGA demonstrated random scission mode under normal conditions (i.e. in water or phosphate buffer medium of pH 7.4 at 37 °C), while unzipping mode (chain-end scission) under harsh conditions (such as high acidity, high temperature, or high energy radiation).[50] Clearly, this complex degradation process indicates the difficulties in controlling the release rate.

The degradation rate of these polymers, such as PGA, PLA, and PLGA, even can be tailored to satisfy the requirements from several weeks to several years by altering the ratio of polylactic to polyglycolic acid, molecular weight, molecular weight distribution, crystallinity, hydrophilicity, pH of the surrounding fluids, as well as specimen size, geometry, porosity, surface properties and sterilization methods.[51] The degradation rate becomes slower as the molecular weight becomes higher. The lower the crystallinity, the higher is the chance of penetration of water molecules to initiate hydrolysis of the chains. Gamma irradiation used for sterilization at doses of 2-3 MRad can result in significant backbone degradation since aliphatic polymers are sensitive to radiation damage. These materials are usually sterilized by exposure to ethylene oxide. Unfortunately, the use of ethylene oxide gas represents a serious safety hazard as well as potentially leaving residual traces in the polymeric devices. They must be degassed for extended periods of time.

Polymer crystallinity is a measure of the alignment of polymeric chains along each other. The presence of bulky side groups, branches and freely mobile atoms (like oxygen in the backbone bonds) adversely influences the alignment of neighboring chains and thus crystallinity. Because lactic acid has a chiral center, PLA can exist in four stereoisomeric forms, poly(L-lactic acid), poly(D-lactic acid), meso-poly(DL-lactic acid), and the racemic mixture of poly(L-lactic acid) and poly(D-lactic acid). Steroregular poly(L-lactic acid) is semicrystalline, while the racemic poly(DL-lactic acid) is amorphous.

In the same conditions, hydrophilic PGA degrades faster in aqueous solutions or *in vivo* than the hydrophobic PLA because the adsorption of water molecules is higher into the chain of the former polymer, although the ester bonds in them have about the same chemical reactivity towards water. The extra methyl group in the PLA repeating unit (compared with PGA) makes it more hydrophobic, reduces the molecular affinity to water, and thus leading to a slower hydrolysis rate. Therefore, it seems that the higher the glycolic acid content, the faster the degradation rate. However, the lifetime of PLGA becomes shortest at PLA/PGA ratio of 50/50, because the more crystalline domains of PGA form as the amount of glycolic acid in the copolymer increases.[52] In the crystalline state, the polymer chains are densely packed and organized to resist the penetration of water. Consequently, backbone hydrolysis tends to only occur at the surface of the crystalline regions, which takes a much longer time than hydrolysis in amorphous polymer or in the amorphous regions of a semicrystalline polymer.

The mechanical properties of biodegradable polymers depend on its chemical structure, crystallinity, molecular weight, or molecular orientation. Table 4 highlights the mechanical properties of selected biodegradable polymers.[9,12,53,54]

Clearly, degradation leads to a loss of mechanical properties and an increase in crystallinity as a result of content loss. PGA loses mechanical integrity between two and four weeks while PLA takes many months or even years to lose mechanical integrity *in vitro* or *in vivo*.[55,56] The amorphous regions of semicrystalline polymers are subjected to degradation earlier than the crystalline regions, leading to an increase in crystallinity. Heterogeneity index (HI, M_w/M_n), an indicator of molecular weight distribution, increases upon PLGA degradation, indicating a faster decrease in M_n (number average molecular weight) in comparison to a decrease in M_w (weight average molecular weight).

Table 4. Mechanical properties of selected biodegradable polymers.

Polymers	Elastic Modulus (GPa)	Tensile Strength (MPa)	Ultimate Elongation (%)
PGA(polyglycolide)	>6.9	>68.9	15-20
PLLA(semicrystalline)	2.4-4.2	55.2-82.7	5-10
PDLLA(amorphous)	1.4-2.8	27.6-41.4	3-10
PLGA	1.4-2.08	41.4-55.2	3-10
PCL(poly(ε-caprolactone))	0.21-0.34	20.7-34.5	300-500

There are other aliphatic polyesters, such as poly(ε-caprolactone) (PCL), which is also used in bone tissue engineering applications.[57] PCL degrades at a significantly slower rate than PLA, PGA, and PLGA[58-60]. A slow degradation rate makes PCL less attractive for general tissue engineering applications, but more attractive for long-term implants and controlled drug release applications. PCL-based copolymers have recently been synthesized to improve degradation properties.[61] Poly(propylene fumarate) (PPF) is also an important synthetic biodegradable polymer and can degrade through hydrolysis of the ester bonds similar to glycolide and lactide polymers.[62] The mechanical properties of PPF can vary greatly according to the synthesis method and the cross-linking agents used.[63]

Naturally derived polymers, such as collagen, have also been used for scaffold fabrication.[64-66] Collagen is a fibrous protein and a major natural extracellular matrix component. On one hand, collagen (as the most popular natural polymer for tissue regeneration by far) has very attractive biological properties (such as biocompatibility) desirable for bone tissue engineering applications; on the other hand, there are concerns over collagen because of poor handling and poor mechanical properties to support bone loading requirements. Denatured collagen (gelatin) has also been processed into porous materials for bone tissue repair.[67-69] To increase the strength of these natural materials, they are often combined with ceramics.[70]

4.2.2. Bioactive Ceramics

The main advantage of using ceramics lies in their high cytocompatibility with bone cells. For bone tissue engineering, alumina, zirconia, titania, and calcium phosphates (such as calcium tetraphosphate ($Ca_4P_2O_9$), tricalcium phosphate (TCP, $Ca_3(PO_4)_2$), hydroxyapatite (HA, $Ca_{10}(PO_4)_6(OH)_2$) and its derivatives, as well as their combinations) are the most common types of bioceramics that have been used to fabricate scaffolds for bone tissue regeneration.[71,72] These ceramics are widely considered to be osteoconductive because their surface properties support osteoblast adhesion, growth, and differentiation and are also reported to be osteoinductive as a result of their capacity to bind and concentrate bone morphogenetic proteins (BMPs) *in vivo*.[73] Moreover, selected ceramics, such as HA and TCP, due to their chemical and structural similarity to the mineral phase of native bone, can react with physiological fluids and form tenacious bonds to hard and soft tissues through cellular activity, thus classifying them as "bioactive".[74,75] In addition, the dissolution rate of HA depends on its crystallinity, and therefore, it can be controlled to be compatible with the rate of new bone growth. The dissolution of HA crystals has been observed to be much slower than amorphous HA.[76]

Due to their excellent bioactivity, these ceramics are often used as coating materials to modify surfaces of traditional metal implants for the purpose of improved bonding to juxtaposed bone (i.e. osseointegration). Various techniques, such as sputtering, electron beam deposition, and plasma spraying, have been used to deposit calcium phosphate and HA on metal substrates. So far, plasma spraying has been most widely used and commercialized because of its simplicity and cost effectiveness. Regardless of the coating technique, the amorphous HA coating generally has a high dissolution rate in aqueous solution than crystalline HA coating. Although the biocompatibility of metal implants can be improved using bioactive ceramic coating, the intrinsic problems of metallic implants (such as much higher stiffness than bone) still can not be solved by these coating methods.

The clinical applications of these bioactive ceramics in large bone defects repair have been limited because of their intrinsic brittleness, difficulty in deforming and shaping, and poor mechanical properties preventing them sustain the mechanical loading needed for bone remodeling.

4.2.3. Ceramic/Polymer Biocomposites

The design of ceramic/polymer composites offers an exceptional approach to combine the advantages of bioactive ceramics and biodegradable polymers to optimize physical, mechanical, and biological properties of scaffolds for bone regeneration. In the past few years, the development of ceramic/polymer composites as scaffold materials for bone tissue engineering has attracted more and more attention.[38,77,78]

First, in ceramic/polymer composites, osteoblast functions can be enhanced from better cell seeding and growth environments due to improved osteoconductivity properties provided by the bioactive ceramic phase.[79-83] For example, Ma et al. prepared highly porous PLA/HA composite scaffolds with a thermal-induced phase separation technique and demonstrated that osteoblast survival percentages and proliferation rates in the PLA/HA scaffolds were higher than in the pure PLA scaffolds.[83]

Second, ceramic particles (such as Bioglass®, HA and TCP) used as inclusions in biodegradable polyesters can provide a pH buffering effect at the polymer surface and tailor the desired degradation and resorption kinetics of the polymer matrix; thus, preventing acceleration of polymer degradation, avoiding the formation of an unfavorable environment for the cells, and reducing side-effects (such as inflammation) from acidic degradation by-products.[38]

Third, the stiffer particulate ceramic phase in polymer composites is important for improving scaffold mechanical properties.[84-87] The addition of biodegradable polymers such as PLA, PGA, and PLGA to calcium phosphate ceramics would allow for better manipulation and control over both the macro- and microstructure in shaping composites to fit bone defects. Furthermore, biodegradable polymers can be used as binders for HA or TCP to reduce the brittleness of the ceramics.[88,89] For example, Thomson et al. demonstrated that the compressive yield strength increased from 0.95 ± 0.11 MPa for PLGA foams to 2.82 ± 0.63 MPa for foams with PLGA/HA fiber weight ratios of 7/6.[78] Moreover, Marra et al. reported that the Young's modulus increased from 2.5 ± 0.7 MPa to 12.5 ± 3.2 MPa when 10 wt. % HA was incorporated into a PCL/PLGA blend with a weight ratio of 10/90.[80] Wei et al. have also demonstrated that the compressive modulus of HA/PLA scaffolds increased with HA content.[17] Specifically, the modulus increased from 4.3 MPa for the plain PLA scaffolds to 8.3 MPa when the weight ratio of HA to PLA was 50/50.[17]

These ceramic/polymer biocomposites demonstrated many promising advantages over traditional single phase materials for orthopedic applications; however, they are still not ideal because they can not mimic many aspects of natural bone, especially nano-scale features of bone.

5. Nanocomposites: Next-Generation Materials in Orthopedics

5.1. Rationale and Evidence

As mentioned, natural bone is a nanostructured composite composed of a polymer matrix (mainly collagen) reinforced with nanometer-sized ceramic particles (mainly carbonated HA). Recent researches in bone regeneration suggested that better osteoconductivity would be achieved if synthetic materials were fabricated to resemble bone in terms of its nano-scale features.[90,91] For example, Du et al. synthesized nano-HA/collagen composites with a porous microstructure similar to bone and these materials promoted the deposition of a new bone matrix. Furthermore, they showed that osteoblasts within this biologically-inspired composite eventually acquired a three-dimensional polygonal shape that integrated with juxtaposed bone fragments.[90,91]

Moreover, nano-sized HA in bone has other special properties due to its small size and huge specific surface area. Specifically, Webster et al. reported significant increase in initial protein adsorption and subsequent osteoblast adhesion on the nano-sized ceramic materials compared to respective traditional micron-sized ceramic materials (such as HA, titania, and alumina).[92-94] Scaffold materials with surface properties similar to physiological bone (characterized by surface grain sizes in the nanometer regime) would aid in the formation of new bone at the tissue/biomaterial interface.[95] Therefore, it is clear that one approach for the design of next generation scaffold materials should incorporate nano-dimensional structures in an effort to mimic natural bone.

Orthopedic implants with surface properties that promote cell and tissue interactions that lead to implant osseointegration are needed. Surface properties such as area, charge and topography depend on the grain size of a material; in this respect, nanophase materials, which, by their very nature, possess higher surface area with increased portions of surface defects such as edge-corner sites and grain boundaries, have an advantage that currently remains largely unexplored for biomedical applications. Surface roughness determined by grain size, crystallinity, and microporosity influence interactions (such as adsorption and/or configuration or bioactivity) of select proteins and subsequent cell adhesion.[92,96,97] Liu et al reported that nanophase titania/PLGA composites which had closest surface roughness to natural bone demonstrated greatest osteoblast adhesion and subsequent calcium-containing mineral deposition.[98] Wei et al. demonstrated greater initial protein adsorption important for osteoblast adhesion on nano-HA/PLA porous scaffolds than on respective micro-HA/PLA scaffolds.[17]

Few studies have addressed the mechanisms of enhanced osteoblast activity on nanophase materials. One set of *in vitro* studies pinpoints grain size in the nanometer regime as the major parameter for enhancing ceramic cytocompatibility. For example, compared to respective conventional, larger grain size, ceramic formulations, enhanced adhesion of osteoblasts and decreased adhesion of fibroblasts (cells that contribute to fibrous encapsulation and callus formation events that may lead to implant loosening and failure) have been observed on nanophase alumina, titania, and HA.[92] In fact, decreasing alumina grain size from 167 to 24 nm increased osteoblast adhesion 51% and at the same time decreased fibroblast adhesion 235% after 4 hours.[93]

Investigations of the underlying mechanisms revealed that the concentration, conformation, and bioactivity of vitronectin (a protein contained in serum that is known to mediate osteoblast adhesion) was responsible for the select, enhanced adhesion of osteoblasts (a crucial prerequisite for subsequent, anchorage-dependent-cell functions) on these novel nanophase ceramic formulations. Vitronectin is a linear protein 15 nm in length and preferentially adsorbed to the small pores present in nanophase ceramics, such as 0.98 nm pores for nanophase titania compacts. For example, adsorption of vitronectin was 10% greater on nanophase compared to conventional alumina.[99] Furthermore, protein conformation plays a critical role in mediating subsequent cell interactions. Increased unfolding of vitronectin adsorbed on nanophase ceramics compared to conventional ceramics was observed.[99] Vitronectin unfolding promoted the availability of specific cell-adhesive epitopes (such as the RGD sequence) for subsequent enhanced osteoblast adhesion; evidence supporting this claim was provided by competitive inhibition studies.[99]

Importantly, nanophase biocomposites may be synthesized to possess hardness, bending, compressive and tensile strengths that are significantly different than conventional materials but more similar to those of physiological bone. Indeed, greater mechanical properties have been reported for biocomposites with a reduction in ceramic grain size to nanometer range. McManus et al. reported that the bending moduli of composites of PLA with 40 and 50 wt. % nanophase (< 100 nm) alumina, titania and HA were significantly greater than respective composite formulations with conventional coarser grained ceramics. Specifically, compared to a bending modulus of 60 ± 3 MPa for plain PLA and 870 ± 30 MPa for conventional titania/PLA composites with the weight ratio of 50/50, the bending modulus of nanophase titania/PLA composites with the weight ratio of 50/50 was 1960 ± 250 MPa, which were on the same order of magnitude of healthy trabecular bone.[23]

Mechanical deformation theory indicates that high-volume fraction of interfacial regions compared to bulk materials leads to increased deformation by grain-boundary sliding and short-range diffusion-healing events as grain size is reduced, and thus increased ductility in nanocrystalline ceramics. Compared to conventional ceramics, nanophase ceramics possess increased surface roughness resulting from both decreased grain size and decreased diameter of surface pores. Moreover, nanophase ceramics possess enhanced surface wettability due to greater surface roughness and greater numbers of grain boundaries on their surfaces.

Nanostructured biocomposites provide alternatives not yet fully explored for orthopedic applications. They may be fabricated to possess similar microarchitecture as that of healthy, physiological bone. Their improved mechanical properties and biocompatibility promise improved orthopedic efficacy in the future.

5.2. Fabrication Techniques of Biocomposite Scaffolds

The commonly accepted concept defines nanomaterials as those materials with basic structural units in the range of 1-100 nm (nanostructured), Nanomaterials exhibit enhanced magnetic, catalytic, optical, electrical, and mechanical properties when compared to conventional formulations of the same material.[100-102] However, to date, relative few advantages of nanocomposites have been taken for orthopedic applications due to the limitation of available fabrication techniques. Therefore, it is important to review the promise of fabrication techniques used for making nanostructured bone substitutes or scaffolds.

Biocomposites can be fabricated with different technologies. The selection of the most appropriate manufacturing technology is also influenced by the relatively low volumes of the production and relatively low dominance of the manufacturing cost over the overall cost of the device. In the body, tissues are organized into three-dimensional structures as functional organs and organ systems. To engineer functional tissues and organs successfully, the scaffolds have to be designed to facilitate cell distribution and guide tissue regeneration in three dimensions.

5.2.1. Solvent-Casting/Particulate-Leaching

Solvent-casting/particulate-leaching (SC/PL) technique has been widely used to fabricate 3D porous polymer scaffolds for tissue engineering applications. Salt (Sodium Chloride) is the most commonly used particulate (also called porogen) because it is easily available and very easy to handle. Briefly, this technique involves producing a suspension of polymer composites in a solvent. Salt particles are ground and sieved into small particles and those of the desired size (most researchers used 100-200 μm range paticles) are transferred into a mold. A polymer suspension is then cast into the salt-filled mold. The solvent is then removed by evaporation in air and/or in vacuum. After the evaporation of the solvent, the salt crystals are leached away by immersion in water to form a porous structure, as schematically shown in Fig. 7. In this technique, the pore size can be controlled by the size of the porogen particles and the porosity can be controlled by the salt/polymer composite ratio.

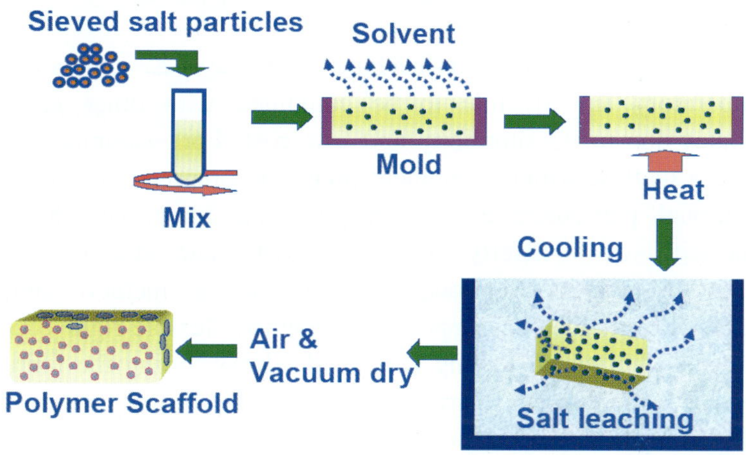

Figure 7. The schematic diagram of solvent-casting particulate-leaching techniques.

Other porogens, such as gelatin, were also studied to replace salt particles. Suh et al. compared the biocompatibility of the two PLGA scaffolds made from either salt porogen (salt scaffold) or gelatin particles (gelatin scaffold) by this technique. Their results demonstrated that the gelatin scaffold showed better attachment of chondrocytes (from knee cartilage) and smooth muscle cells (from bladder) at the initial stage, and both cell types showed much better proliferation of cells during 3 months. Suh et al. believed that the better performance of a gelatin scaffold also contributed to the better connection of pores at the same porosity.[103]

Using waxy hydrocarbons as porogens was also reported in the fabrication of PLA and PLGA scaffolds with up to 87% porosity and pores over 100 μm in diameter.[104] After mixing the waxy hydrocarbon and polymer (dissolved in chloroform) into a paste, the composite was cast into a desired mold. The mold was then immersed in a hydrocarbon solvent (pentane or hexane) to remove the wax without dissolving the PLA or PLGA. The remaining foam was vacuum dried for several days to extract any solvents. Thick samples (up to 2.5 cm) with interconnected pores can be created using this technique. This method also offers the possibility of adding a second phase to the paste to create a composite which could increase the strength or electrical conductivity of the final scaffolds.

Solvent-casting/particulate-leaching technique is easy to carry out in the laboratory and flexible to be combined with other fabrication techniques due to its simplicity and low cost. For example, Wu et al reported a method which combined modified compression molding and conventional particulate-leaching to fabricate complexly shaped 3D porous scaffolds.[105] Briefly, a polymer-particulate mixture was first prepared by the conventional solvent casting method and then compressively molded in a specially designed flexible-rigid combined mold which facilitates shaping and mold release during the fabrication process. The molding was carried out at a moderate temperature, above the glass transition temperature and below the flow temperature of these amorphous polymers. A porous scaffold was then obtained after particulate leaching. Highly interconnected and uniformly distributed pores both in the bulk and on the external surface of the PLA and PLGA auricle-shaped scaffolds were observed, and the porosity could exceed 90%.[105]

However, solvent-casting/particulate-leaching technique has four main disadvantages. First, this technique usually involves organic solvents which are not favorable for tissue engineering applications due to potential harmful influences on cells and tissues. Organic solvents also in many cases preclude the possibility of adding pharmacological agents to the scaffold during the fabrication. Secondly, certain critical variables such as pore shape and inter-pore openings are still not well controlled in this technique. Third, when applying this technique to polymer/ceramic composite scaffolds, the polymer-organic solvent solutions may coat the bioactive ceramic surfaces, hinder their exposure to the scaffold surface, and decrease their direct contact with osteogenic cells which are crucial for osseointegration. The last but not the least, if nanophase ceramic particles were used to make nanocomposite scaffolds in this technique, nanoparticles may interfere the porogen leaching process, which will result in residual porogen particles in the final tissue engineering products, and thus, having adverse effects on their biocompatibility.

5.2.2. Gas-Foaming/Particulate-Leaching

Due to the problems associated with the solvent-casting particulate-leaching technique, gas-foaming/particulate-leaching (GF/PL) was proposed by Mooney et al. without the use of organic solvent, as shown in Fig. 8.[106] Disks comprised of polymer (e.g., PLGA) and salt (NaCl) particles were compression molded at room temperature and subsequently allowed to saturate with high pressure carbon dioxide (CO_2) gas (800 psi). The solubility of the gas in the polymer was then decreased rapidly by bringing the CO_2 pressure back to atmospheric level, which created a thermodynamic instability leading to the nucleation and growth of gas pores in the polymer particles, resulting in the expansion of the polymer particles. The polymer particles fused to form a continuous matrix with entrapped salt particles. The NaCl particles subsequently were leached away in water to yield macropores within the polymer matrix. The overall porosity and level of pore connectivity were regulated by the ratio of polymer/salt particles and the size of salt particles. Both the compressive modulus (289 ± 25 kPa versus 159 ± 130 kPa) and the tensile modulus (1100 ± 236 kPa versus 334 ± 52 kPa) of the scaffolds formed with this approach were significantly greater than those formed with a standard solvent casting/particulate leaching process.

Gas-foaming/particulate-leaching technique could be directly applied to fabricate nanophase ceramic/polymer composite scaffolds without major modifications. For example, Kim et al fabricated nano-HA/PLGA composite scaffolds for bone tissue engineering using this technique.[107]

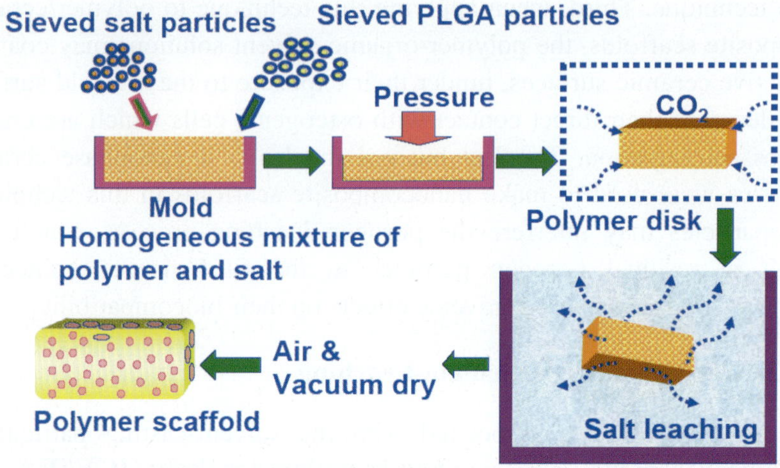

Figure 8. The schematic diagram of the gas-foaming/particulate-leaching technique.

HA particles with approximately 100 nm in size rather than micro-sized particles, were used to fabricate the composite scaffolds to increase the HA exposure to the scaffold surface without increasing the amount of HA. The GF/PL method exposed HA nanoparticles at the scaffold surface significantly more than the conventional SC/PL method does. The GF/PL scaffolds showed interconnected porous structures without a skin layer and exhibited superior enhanced mechanical properties to those of scaffolds fabricated by the SC/PL method. Both types of scaffolds were seeded with rat calvarial osteoblasts and cultured in vitro or were subcutaneously implanted into athymic mice for eight weeks. The GF/PL scaffolds exhibited significantly higher cell growth, alkaline phosphatase activity, and mineralization compared to the SC/PL scaffolds *in vitro*. Histological analyses and calcium content quantification of the regenerated tissues five and eight weeks after implantation showed that bone formation was more extensive on the GF/PL scaffolds than on the SC/PL scaffolds. Compared to the SC/PL scaffolds, the enhanced bone formation on the GF/PL scaffolds may have resulted from the higher exposure of HA nanoparticles at the scaffold surface, which allowed for direct contact with the transplanted cells and stimulated the cell proliferation and osteogenic differentiation.

However, the both SC/PL and GF/PL techniques have limited range of pore sizes (i.e., 100-500 μm) in the composite scaffolds, as shown in Fig. 9.[107]

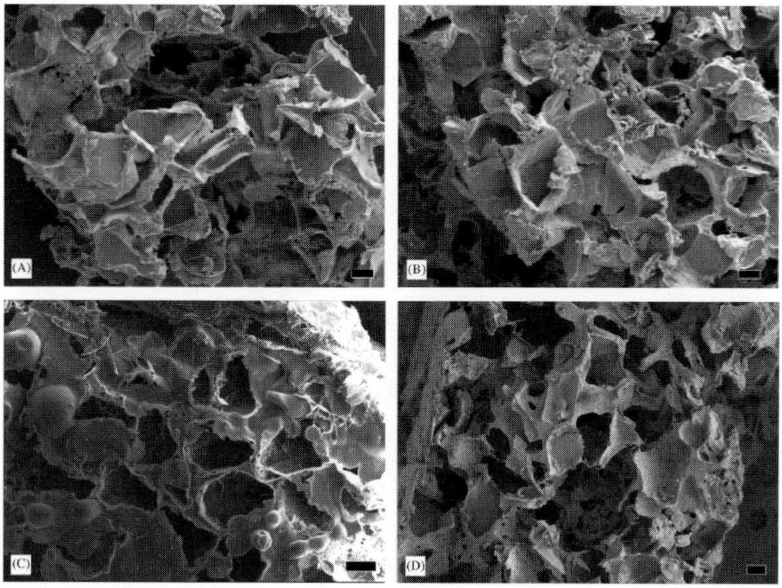

Figure 9. Scanning electron micrographs of (A,C) surfaces and (B,D) cross-sections of the nano-HA/PLGA composite scaffolds fabricated by (A,B) the SC/PL method and (C,D) the GF/PL method. The scale bars indicate 100 μm.

Modified gas-foaming technique using gas foaming salt such as ammonium bicarbonate instead of CO_2 was reported by Nam et al., as shown in Fig. 10.[108] Ammonium bicarbonate was added to a polymer solution to obtain a highly viscous mixture, which could be shaped by hand or using a mold. The solvent was then evaporated and the composite was either vacuum dried or immersed in warm water. Vacuum drying caused the ammonium bicarbonate to sublime while immersion in water resulted in concurrent gas evolution and particle leaching. The latter method wass preferred because it did not result in the creation of a nonporous outer skin, as seen in the vacuum-dried scaffolds. Porosities as high as 90% with pore sizes from 200-500 μm were attained using this technique.

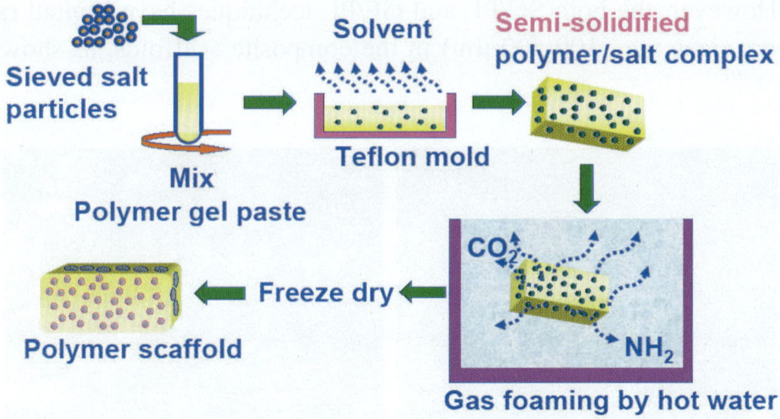

Figure 10. The schematic diagram of gas foaming using ammonium bicarbonate.

5.2.3. Phase Separation and Emulsion Freeze Drying

A homogeneous multi-component system, under certain conditions, becomes thermodynamically unstable and tends to separate into more than one phase in order to lower the system free energy, which is called phase separation. Based on this principle, solid-liquid phase separation (Fig. 11) and liquid-liquid phase separation (Fig. 12) were developed for the fabrication of 3D porous scaffolds.

Solid-liquid phase separation, also called emulsion freeze drying, could be achieved by lowering the temperature to induce solvent crystallization from a polymer suspension (solid phase formation in a liquid phase). After the removal of the solvent crystals (sublimation or solvent exchange), the space originally taken by the solvent crystals becomes pores.[109] As an example, PLGA was first dissolved in chloroform and then distilled water was added. The polymer, organic solvent, and water were mixed by a stirrer to form an emulsion and the emulsion was then cast into a mold and quenched by placing in liquid nitrogen to solidify the mixture and induce solid-liquid phase separation. After quenching, the scaffolds were lyophilized (freeze-dried) at -55°C, resulting in the removal of the dispersed water and polymer solvents. The scaffolds made by this technique had large porosities (91-95%), and small median pore size (13-35 μm) with large pore size distribution

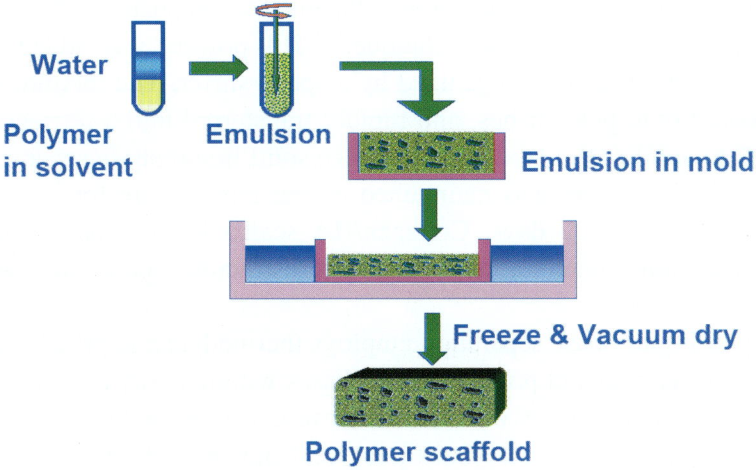

Figure 11. The schematic diagram of solid-liquid phase separation.

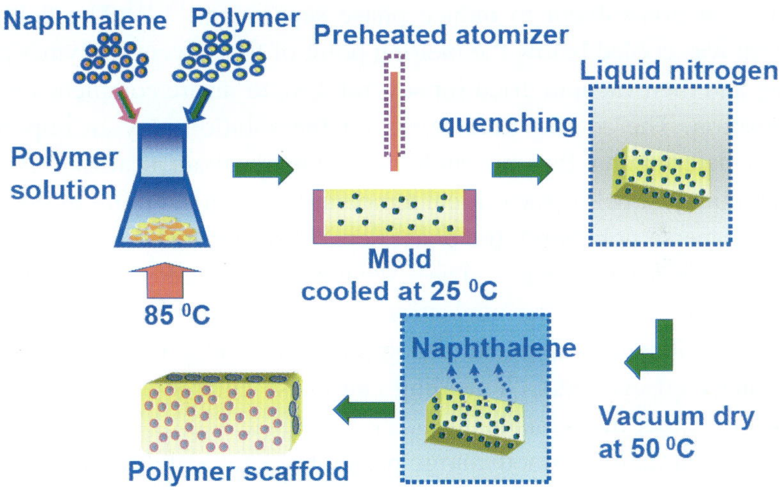

Figure 12. The schematic diagram of liquid-liquid phase separation.

(larger pore diameters greater than 200 μm).[109] Various pore structures can be achieved by varying processing parameters such as water volume fraction in polymer solution, polymer weight percentage, polymer molecular weight and viscosity of the emulsion.

Furthermore, Liu et al. prepared collagen/HA composite scaffolds by solid-liquid phase separation technique.[110] HA powder was added into collagen solution, and homogenized by a speed stirrer. The mixture was then poured onto petri dishes, and rapidly transferred into a refrigerator at -30°C to solidify the mixture and induce solid-liquid phase separation. The solidified mixture was maintained at that temperature for 2 h, and then lyophilized for 2 days. Collagen/HA scaffolds were porous with three-dimension interconnected fiber microstructure, pore size were 50-150 μm.

Liquid-liquid phase separation employs thermodynamic principles to create polymer-rich and polymer-poor phases within a polymer solution. The polymer poor phase was then removed, leaving a highly porous polymer network. Both PLA and PLGA scaffolds have been formulated using this technique.[111-113] The polymers were dissolved in a solvent with a low melting point and that was easy to sublime, such as naphthalene, phenol or 1,4 dioxane. In some cases, small amounts of water were added as a non-solvent to induce phase separation.[113, 114] The polymer solution was cooled below the melting point of the solvent (polymer poor phase) and then vacuum dried for several days to insure complete solvent sublimation. The cooling parameters for the solution play an important role in determining the morphology of the resultant scaffold. At the temperature just below the critical temperature (or cloud point in the case of polydisperse polymers), the phase separation occured via a nucleation and growth mechanism. The separation occured via spinodal decomposition. While the nucleation and growth mechanism results in spheroidal domains, spinodal decomposition causes the formation of interconnected cylinders. Annealing can cause enlargement of domains formed by either mechanism.

Based on these thermodynamic principles, spinodal decomposition is preferred as it increases the number of interconnected pores within the network.[113-114] In addition, it has been found that annealing is important to increase pore size. Various parameters that influence the phase diagram of the system, and thus the resulting pore morphology, are polymer concentration, cooling method and time, solvent/nonsolvent ratio, and the presence of surfactants, which can reduce the interfacial tension between phases and increase pore size and interconnectivity. Various parameters can be changed to tailor pore size and porosity for specific applications is appealing.

This technique can be used to fabricate scaffolds from many types of polymers and polymeric composite materials. However, although this technique is advantageous as it does not require an extra washing/leaching step, the use of organic solvents remains a concern for the inclusion of cells and bioactive molecules. Moreover, the phase diagrams of the polymer-solvent systems must be better characterized before this flexibility can be fully exploited for use in tissue-engineered constructs. The pores formed using phase separation techniques usually have diameters on the order of a few to tens of microns and are often not uniformly distributed.

This indicates that this fabrication method currently has limited usefulness in the field of tissue engineering. Controlled phase separation processes, primarily thermally induced phase separation, have also been explored for scaffold fabrication. [114]

5.2.4. Fiber Meshes/Fiber Bonding

Fibers, produced by textile technology, have been used to make non-woven scaffolds from PGA and PLLA. The lack of structural stability of these nonwoven scaffolds, often resulted in significant deformation due to contractile forces of the cells that have been seeded on the scaffold. This led to the development of a fiber bonding technique to increase the mechanical properties of the scaffolds. This is achieved by dissolving PLLA in methylene chloride and casting over the PGA mesh. The solvent is allowed to evaporate and the construct is then heated above the melting point of PGA. Once the PGA-PLLA construct has cooled, the PLLA is removed by dissolving in methylene chloride again. This treatment results in a mesh of PGA fibers joined at the cross-points.

5.2.5. Melt Molding

This process involves filling a Teflon mould with PLGA powder and gelatine microspheres, of specific diameter, and then heating the mould above the glass-transition temperature of PLGA while applying pressure to the mixture. This treatment causes the PLGA particles to bond together. Once the mould is removed, the gelatin component is leached out by immersing in water and the scaffold is then dried. Scaffolds produced this way assume the shape of the mould. The melt molding process was modified to incorporate short fibers of HA. A uniform distribution of HA fibers throughout the PLGA scaffold could only be accomplished by using a solvent-casting technique to prepare a composite material of HA fibres, PLGA matrix and gelatine or salt porogen, which was then used in the melt moulding process.

5.2.6. Freeze Drying and Cross-linking

Kim et al. reported that hydroxyapatite (HA) and gelatin composites were fabricated in a foam type via a novel freeze-drying and cross-linking technique. The HA powder was added at up to 30 wt% into the gelatin solution, and the mixtures were freeze-dried and further crosslinked. The pure gelatin foam had a well-developed pore configuration with porosity and pore size of ~90% and 400-500 μm, respectively. With HA addition, the porosity decreased and pore shape became more irregular. The HA particulates, in sizes of about 2-5 μm, were distributed within the gelatin network homogeneously and made the framework surface rougher. All the foams had high water absorption capacities, showing typical hydrogel characteristics, even though the HA addition decreased the degree of water absorption. The HA addition made the foam much stronger and stiffer, i.e., with increasing HA amount the foams sustained higher compressive stress and had higher elastic modulus in both dry and wet states.

5.2.7. Rapid Prototyping Techniques

One of the common shortcomings of the fabrication technologies discussed above is the lack of precise control of the three-dimensional pore architecture of the scaffolds. To tackle this problem, solid free form fabrication (also known as rapid prototyping) techniques are being adopted. The main advantage of these techniques is their ability to produce complex-shaped objects rapidly from a computer-aided design (CAD) model. One of these rapid prototyping techniques, called 3D printing, was first developed at the Massachusetts Institute of Technology and has been used to process biodegradable polymer scaffolds for tissue engineering applications. This process generates components by ink-jet printing a binder on to sequential powder layers. The operation parameters such as the speed, flow rate, and drop position can be computer controlled to produce complex 3D polymer scaffolds. Biological agents, such as growth factors, can also be incorporated into the scaffolds in the printing process. However, rapid prototyping techniques have inherent shortcomings such as limited material selection and inadequate resolution. The resolution is determined by the size of binder drops, the jet and powder particles, which makes it difficult to design and fabricate scaffolds with fine microstructures. The porosity of the scaffold fabricated with this method is low, and the mechanical properties of the scaffolds have to be significantly improved. Similarly, other rapid prototyping techniques, such as fused deposition modeling (FDM) and stereolithography have also been explored for composite fabrication.

Three-dimensional ink-writing techniques can be divided into two approaches: (1) droplet-based or (2) continuous (filamentary) inks. Three-dimensional periodic structures offer the greatest challenge for designing inks, because they contain self-supporting (or spanning) features. Inks are typically formulated from colloidal, polymeric, or polyelectrolyte building blocks suspended or dissolved in a liquid or heated to create a stable, homogeneous ink with the desired and reproducible rheological (or flow) behavior. The important rheological parameters for a given ink design include its apparent viscosity, yield stress under shear and compression, and viscoelastic properties (i.e. the shear loss and elastic moduli), which are tailored for the specific direct-write technique of interest. Three-dimensional printing (3DP), direct ink-jet printing, and related approaches such as hot-melt printing, involve patterning materials using an ink-jet print head, similar to those used in desktop document printing. These approaches require either low viscosity fluids that must be removed by absorption and evaporation or wax-based inks that are heated during droplet formation and then solidify upon impact cooling. Cima and Sachs pioneered the concept of using ink-jet printing (3DP) to assemble materials. In 3DP, low viscosity binder droplets are printed onto a powder bed to locally "fuse" material together in a desired pattern. After defining a given two-dimensional layer, an additional powder layer is spread across the bed surface and subsequently patterned. In other ink-jet approaches, three-dimensional structures, such as high-aspect ratio walls or concentrated nanoparticle inks; however, clogging issues still arise when D/2 a~150, where D is the finest nozzle used (30 μm in diameter) and a is the radius of largest ink particles. These three-dimensional mesoscale structures may find potential application as tissue engineering scaffolds, if constructed from a bioactive ceramic material (e.g. hydroxyapatite), or as structural or functional composites, if the pore space is filled with a second phase.

In addition, the resulting constructs have structural heterogeneity because of the "pixel assembly" nature of the rapid prototyping fabrication process. To overcome this shortcoming, a reverse fabrication technique has been developed to fabricate a negative replica of the scaffold. A polymer/ceramic suspension is cast into such a mold and solidified after the removal of the solvent. The mold is then dissolved away to form the scaffold with the designed three-dimensional pore network. The scaffold is more homogeneous, but the feature resolution is not improved.

To achieve higher resolution for scaffolds with well-controlled interconnected spherical pores, paraffin spheres are fabricated by a dispersion method. These paraffin spheres are then transferred into a three-dimensional mold of the designed shape. The spheres are bonded together through a heat treatment process. A composite suspension is cast into the paraffin assembly in the mold. After removal of the solvent, the paraffin sphere assembly is dissolved away. In this way, an interconnected spherical pore structure is created. Importantly, the features generated have significantly better resolution than those achievable with current rapid prototyping techniques. In addition, investment in expensive equipment is not required, which allows the technology to be easily adapted to a research, as well as an industrial, setting.

5.3. Future Directions in Orthopedics

Simply stated, there are a number of future directions for the use of nanoceramic polymer composites:

1) Improve fabrication techniques of polymer/ceramic composites, including resolution and preciseness of three-dimensional structures.
2) Improve mechanical properties closer to natural tissue, such as strength and elastic modulus of polymer/ceramic composites. Improve biocompatibility, particularly long-term cell functions on synthesized biocomposites.
3) Study degradation behavior of biodegradable polymer and bioactive ceramic composites, specially the effect of ceramic phase on degradation kinetics and degradation product.
4) Incorporate drugs and growth factor into biocomposite scaffolds.
5) Modify composites surface to favor cell growth and improve composite-tissue interface.

Bibliography

1. Smith R. (2004) *Bone Health and Osteoporosis: A Report of the Surgeon General*, U.S. Department of Health and Human Services, Public Health Service, Office of the Surgeon General, Rockville, MD, pp. 68-70, 2004.
2. Bren L (2004) *Joint replacement: an inside look.* FDA Consumer, 38(2). http://www.fda.gov/fdac/features/2004/204_joints.html
3. Webster TJ. (2003) Nanophase ceramics as improved bone tissue engineering materials. *American Ceramic Society Bulletin* **82(6)**: 23-28.
4. Rho JY, Kuhn-Spearing L, and Zioupos P. (1998) Mechanical properties and the hierarchical structure of bone. *Medical Engineering & Physics* **20**: 92-102.
5. Kaplan FS, Hayes WC, Keaveny TM, Boskey A, Einhorn TA, and Iannotti J. (1994) Form and function of bone. In: *Orthopaedic Basic Science*, Simon SR, (ed.), American Academy of Orthopaedic Surgeons, Columbus, OH, pp. 127-185.
6. Webster TJ. (2001) Nanophase ceramics: The future orthopedic and dental implant material. In: *Advances in Chemical Engineering*, Vol. 27, Nanostructured Materials, Ying JY (ed.), Academic Press, San Diego, CA, pp. 126-160.
7. Kuhn-Spearing L, Rey C, Kim HM, and Glimcher MJ. (1996) Carbonated apatite nanocrystals of bone. In: *Synthesis and processing of nanocrystalline powder*, Bourell DL (ed.), The Minerals, Metals and Materials Society, Warrendale, PA, USA.

8. Giraud-Guille MM. (1998) Twisted plywood architecture of collagen fibrils in human compact bone osteons. *Calcified tissue international* **42(3)**: 167–180.
9. Bronzino JD. (2000) *The Biomedical Engineering Handbook*, CRC Press, Boca Raton, FL: pp. 274-706.
10. Black J, and Hastings G. (1998) *Handbook of Biomaterial Properties*, Chapman & Hall, New York, NY, pp. 3-21.
11. Fung YC. (1993) *Biomechanics: Mechanical Properties of Living Tissues*, Springer-Verlag, New York, NY, pp. 500-519.
12. Boccaccini AR, and Blaker JJ. (2005) Bioactive composite materials for tissue engineering scaffolds. *Expert Review of Medical Devices*, **2(3)**: 303-317.
13. Guyton AC. (1991) *Textbook of Medical Physiology*, Saunders, Philadelphia, PA, pp. 868-881.
14. Marin BR, and Burr DB (1989) *Structure Function and Adaptation of Compact Bone*, Raven Press, New York, NY, pp. 106-107.
15. Trippel SB. (1998) Potential role of insulin like growth factors in fracture healing. *Clinical Orthopaedics and Related Research* **355S**: S301-313.
16. Stein GS, Lian JB. (1993) Molecular mechanisms mediating proliferation/ differentiation interrelationships during progressive development of osteoblast phenotype. *Endocrine Reviews* **14(4)**: 424-442.
17. Wei G. and Ma PX. (2004) Structure and properties of nano-hydroxyapatite/ polymer composite scaffolds for bone tissue engineering. *Biomaterials* **25(19)**: 4749-4757.
18. Salgado AJ, Coutinho OP, and Reis RL. (2004) Bone tissue engineering: state of the art and future trends. *Macromolecular Bioscience* **4(8)**: 743-765.
19. Saltzman, WM. (2004) *Tissue Engineering*, Oxford University Press, New York, NY, pp. 6-7.
20. Marra KG, Szem JW, Kumta PN, DiMilla PA, and Weiss LE. (1999) *In vitro* analysis of biodegradable polymer blend/hydroxyapatite composites for bone tissue engineering. *Journal of Biomedical Materials Research*, **47(3)**: 324-335.
21. Nather A. (2003) Biology of healing of large deep-frozen cortical bone allografts. In: *Bone Biology and Healing* Phillips GO (ed.), pp. 50-65.
22. Park JB, and Bronzino JD. (2003) *Biomaterials: Principles and Applications*, CRC Press,, Boca Raton, FL, pp. 1-20.
23. McManus AJ, Doremus RH, Siegel RW, and Bizios R. (2005) Evaluation of cytocompatibility and bending modulus of nanoceramic/polymer composites. *Journal of Biomedical Materials Research* **72A(1)**: 98-106.
24. Skalak R and Fox CF. (1988) *Tissue Engineering: Proceedings of a Workshop Held at Granlibakken, Lake Tahoe, CA*, Alan R Liss., New York, pp. 26-29.
25. Mooney DJ, and Mikos AG. (1999) Growing new organs. *Scientific American*, **280(4)**: 60-65.

26. Sachlos E. and Caernuszka JT. (2003) Making tissue engineering scaffolds work: review on the application of solid free form fabrication technology to the production of tissue engineering scaffolds. *European Cells and Materials* **5**: 29-40.
27. Temenoff JS, Steinbis ES, and Mikos AG. (2004) Biodegradable scaffolds. In: *Orthopedic Tissue Engineering: Basic Science and Practice* Goldberg VM and Caplan AI (eds), Marcel Dekker, New York, pp. 77-95.
28. Leong KF, Cheah CM, and Chua CK. (2003) Solid freeform fabrication of three-dimensional scaffolds for engineering replacement tissues and organs. *Biomaterials*, **24(13)**: 2363-2378.
29. Davies JE. (1996) *In vitro* modeling of the bone/implant interface. *The Anatomical Record* **245(2)**: 426-445.
30. Albrektsson T and Johansson C. (2001) Osteoinduction, osteoconduction and osseointegration. *European Spine Journal*, **10(Supply 2)**: S96-101.
31. Kirker-Head CA. (2000) Potential applications and delivery strategies for bone morphogenetic proteins. *Advanced Drug Delivery Reviews*, **43(1)**: 65-92.
32. Silver, FH (1994) *Biomaterials Medical Devices and Tissue Engineering: An Integrated Approach*, Chapman & Hall, New York, pp. 4-29.
33. Park JB and Bronzino JD (2003) *Biomaterials: Principles and Applications*, CRC Press, Boca Raton, FL, pp. 20-77.
34. Reis RL and Cohn D. (2001) *Polymer Based Systems on Tissue Engineering, Replacement and Regeneration*, Kluwer Academic Publishers, Boston, pp. 69-92,130.
35. Porter BD, Oldham JB, He SL, Zobitz ME, Payne RG, An KN, Currier BL, Mikos AG, and Yaszemski MJ. (2000) Mechanical properties of a biodegradable bone regeneration scaffold. *Transactions of the ASME. Journal of Biomechanical Engineering* **122(3)**: 286-288.
36. Agrawal CM, and Ray RB. (2001) Biodegradable polymeric scaffolds for musculoskeletal tissue engineering. *Journal of Biomedical Materials Research*, **55(2)**: 141-150.
37. Thomson RC, Mikos AG, Beahm E, Lemon JC, Satterfield WC, Aufdemorte TB, and Miller MJ. (1999) Guided tissue fabrication from periosteum using preformed biodegradable polymer scaffolds. *Biomaterials* **20(21)**: 2007-2018.
38. Boccaccini AR, and Maquet V. (2003) Bioresorbable and bioactive polymer/bioglass® composites with tailored pore structure for tissue engineering applications. *Composites Science and Technology*, **63(16)**: 2417-2429.
39. Liu X. and Ma P.X. (2004) Polymeric scaffolds for bone tissue engineering. *Annals of Biomedical Engineering* **32(3)**: 477-486.
40. Chen VJ, and Ma PX (2004) Nano-fibrous poly(L-lactic acid) scaffolds with interconnected spherical macropores. *Biomaterials* **25(11)**: 2065-2073.
41. Karp, JM, Shoichet MS, and Davies JE. (2003) Bone formation on two-dimensional poly(DL-lactide-co-glycolide) (PLGA) films and three-dimensional

PLGA tissue engineering scaffolds *in vitro*. *Journal of Biomedical Materials Research - Part A* **64(2)**: 388-396.

42. Liu X, and Ma PX (2004) Polymeric scaffolds for bone tissue engineering. *Annals of Biomedical Engineering* **32(3)**: 477-486.
43. Gilding DK and Reed AM. (1979) Biodegradable polymers for use in surgery---polyglycolic/poly(lactic acid) homo- and copolymers. *Polymer* **20(12)**: 1459-1464.
44. Rokkanen P, Bostman O, Vainionpaa S, Vihtonen K, Tormala P, Laiho J, Kilpikari J, and Tamminmaki M. (1985) Biodegradable implants in fracture fixation: early results of treatment of fractures of the ankle. *Lancet* **1(8443)**: 1422-1424.
45. Waris E, Konttinen YT, Ashammakhi N, Suuronen R, and Santavirta S. (2004) Bioabsorbable fixation devices in trauma and bone surgery: current clinical standing. *Expert Review of Medical Devices* **1(2)**: 229-240.
46. Gunatillake PA, and Adhikari R. (2003) Biodegradable synthetic polymers for tissue engineering. *European Cells and Materials* **5**: 1-16.
47. Kohn J, Abramson S, and Langer R. (2004) Bioresorbable and bioerodible materials. In *Biomaterials Science: an Introduction to Materials in Medicine* Ratner BD (ed.) Elsevier Academic Press, Boston, MA, pp. 115-126.
48. Cooper SL, Visser SA, Hergenrother RW, and Lamba NMK (2004) Polymers. In: *Biomaterials Science: an Introduction to Materials in Medicine* Ratner BD (ed.) Elsevier Academic Press, Boston, MA, pp. 67-79.
49. Hasirci V. (2000) Biodegradable biomedical polymers: Review of degradation of and *in vivo* response to polylactides and polyhydroxyalkanoates. In: *Biomaterials and Bioengineering Handbook* Wise DL (ed.), Marcel Dekker, New York, NY, pp. 141-155.
50. Shih C. (1995) A graphical method for the determination of the mode of hydrolysis of biodegradable polymers. *Pharmaceutical Research* **12(12)**: 2036-2060.
51. Taddei P, Monti P, and Simoni R. (2002) Vibrational and thermal study on the *in vitro* and *in vivo* degradation of a poly(lactic acid)-based bioabsorbable periodontal membrane. *Journal of Materials Science: Materials in Medicine* **13(5)**: 469-475.
52. Park JB and Bronzino JD (2003) *Biomaterials: Principles and Applications*, CRC Press, Boca Raton, FL, pp. 99-103.
53. Barbucci R. (2002) *Integrated Biomaterials Science*, Kluwer Academic/Plenum Publishers, New York, pp. 189-689.
54. Yang S. Leong KF, Du Z, and Chua CK. (2001) The design of scaffolds for use in tissue engineering. Part 1. traditional factors. *Tissue Engineering* **7(6)**: 679-689.
55. Ma PX and Langer R. (1995) Degradation, structure and properties of fibrous nonwoven poly(glycolic acid) scaffolds for tissue engineering. *Materials Research Society Symposium - Proceedings, Polymers in Medicine and Pharmacy* **394**: 99-104.
56. Zhang R and Ma PX. (2000) Degradation behavior of porous poly(α-hydroxy acids)/hydroxyapatite composite scaffolds. *Polymer Preprints*, published by

Division of Polymer Chemistry Inc. and American Chemical Society, **41(2)**: 1618-1619.

57. Ciapetti G, Ambrosio L, Savarino L, Granchi D, Cenni E, Baldini N, Pagani S, Guizzardi S, Causa F, and Giunti A. (2003) Osteoblast growth and function in porous poly ε-caprolactone matrices for bone repair: a preliminary study. *Biomaterials* **24(21)**: 3815-3824.
58. Pitt CG, Chasalow FI, Hibionada YM, Klimas DM, and Schindler A. (1981) Aliphatic polyesters. I. the degradation of poly(ε-caprolactone) *in vivo*. *Journal of Applied Polymer Science* **26(11)**: 3779-378.
59. Pitt CG, Gratzl MM, Kimmel GL, Surles J, and Schindler A. (1981) Aliphatic polyesters II. the degradation of poly(DL-lactide), poly(ε-caprolactone), and their copolymers *in vivo*. *Biomaterials* **2(4)**: 215-220.
60. Dunn AS, Campbell PG, and Marra KG. (2001) The Influence of polymer blend composition on the degradation of polymer/hydroxyapatite biomaterial. *Journal of Materials Science: Materials in Medicine* **12(8)**: 673-677.
61. Lin W. (1999) Comparison of thermal characteristics and degradation properties of ε-caprolactone copolymers. *Journal of Biomedical Materials Research*: **47**: 420-423.
62. Fisher JP, Vehof JWM, Dean D, Van der Waerden JPCM, Holland TA, Mikos AG, and Jansen JA. (2002) Soft and hard tissue response to photo crosslinked poly(propylene fumarate) scaffolds in a rabbit model. *Journal of Biomedical Materials Research* **59(3)**: 547-556.
63. Temenoff JS and Mikos AG. (2000) Injectable biodegradable materials for orthopedic tissue engineering. *Biomaterials* **21(23)**: 2405-2412.
64. Rodrigues CVM, Serricella P, Linhares ABR, Guerdes RM, Borojevic R, Rossi, MA, Duarte, MEL, and Farina M. (2003) Characterization of a bovine collagen-hydroxyapatite composite scaffold for bone tissue engineering. *Biomaterials* **24(27)**: 4987-4997.
65. Dunn MG, Bellincampi LD, Tria AJ, and Zawadsky JP. (1997) Preliminary development of a collagen-PLA composite for ACL reconstruction. *Journal of Applied Polymer Science* **63(11)**: 1423-1428.
66. Liao SS, Cui FZ, and Zhu Y. (2004) Osteoblasts adherence and migration through three-dimensional porous mineralized collagen based composite: nHAC/PLA. *Journal of Bioactive and Compatible Polymers*, **19(2)**: 117-130.
67. Ren L, Tsuru K, Hayakawa S, and Osaka A (2002) Novel approach to fabricate porous gelatin-siloxane hybrids for bone tissue engineering. *Biomaterials* **23(24)**: 4765-4773.
68. Yin Y, Ye F, Cui J, Zhang F, Li X, and Yao K (2003) Preparation and characterization of macroporous chitosan-gelatin/β-tricalcium phosphate composite scaffolds for bone tissue engineering. *Journal of Biomedical Materials Research - Part A*, **67(3)**: 844-855.

69. Zhao F, Yin Y, Lu WW, Leong JC, Zhang W, Zhang J, Zhang M, and Yao K (2002) Preparation and histological evaluation of biomimetic three-dimensional hydroxyapatite/chitosan-gelatin network composite scaffolds. *Biomaterials* **23(15)**: 3227-3234.
70. Lawson AC and Czernuszka JT. (1998) Collagen-calcium phosphate composites. *Proceedings of the Institution of Mechanical Engineers, Part H: Journal of Engineering in Medicine* **212(H6)**: 413-425.
71. Tadic D, and Epple M. (2004) A thorough physicochemical characterisation of 14 calcium phosphate-based bone substitution materials in comparison to natural bone. *Biomaterials* **25(6)**: 987-994.
72. Ramay HRR and Zhang M. (2004) Biphasic calcium phosphate nanocomposite porous scaffolds for load-bearing bone tissue engineering. *Biomaterials* **25(21)**: 5171-5180.
73. LeGeros RZ Lin S, Rohanizadeh R Mijares D, and Legeros JP. (2003) Biphasic calcium phosphate bioceramics: preparation, properties and applications. *Journal of Materials Science: Materials in Medicine* **14(3)**: 201-209.
74. Hench LL and Polak JM. (2002) Third-generation biomedical materials. *Science* **295(5557)**: 1014-1017.
75. Ducheyne P and de Groot K. (1981) *In vivo* surface activity of a hydroxyapatite alveolar bone substitute. *Journal of Biomedical Materials Research* **15(3)**: 441-445.
76. Rabiei A and Thomas B. (2005) Processing and development of nano-scale HA coating for biomedical application. *Materials Research Society Symposium Proceeding* **845**: 193-199.
77. Hutmacher DW. (2000) Scaffolds in tissue engineering bone and cartilage. *Biomaterials* **21(24)**: 2529-2543.
78. Thomson RC, Yaszemski MJ, Powers JM, and Mikos AG. (1998) Hydroxyapatite fiber reinforced poly(α-hydroxy ester) foams for bone regeneration. *Biomaterials* **19(21)**: 1935-1943.
79. Boccaccini AR, Roether JA, Hench LL, Maquet V, and Jerome R. (2002) A composite approach to tissue engineering. *Ceramic Engineering and Science Proceedings* **23(4)**: 805-816.
80. Marra KG, Szem JW, Kumta PN, DiMilla PA, and Weiss LE. (1999) *In vitro* analysis of biodegradable polymer blend/hydroxyapatite composites for bone tissue engineering. *Journal of Biomedical Materials Research* **47(3)**: 324-335.
81. Kalita S, Finley J, Bose S, Hosick H, and Bandyopadhyay A. (2002) Development of porous polymer-ceramic composites as bone grafts. *Materials Research Society Symposium Proceedings* **726**: 91-96.
82. Blaker JJ, Gough JE, Maquet V, Notingher I, and Boccaccini AR. (2003) *In vitro* evaluation of novel bioactive composites based on bioglass®-filled polylactide foams for bone tissue engineering scaffolds. *Journal of Biomedical Materials Research-Part A* **67(4)**: 1401-1411.

83. Ma PX, Zhang R, Xiao G, and Franceschi R. (2001) Engineering new bone tissue *in vitro* on highly porous poly(α-hydroxyl acids)/hydroxyapatite composite scaffolds. *Journal of Biomedical Materials Research* **54(2)**: 284-293.
84. Kasuga T, Ota Y, Nogami M, and Abe Y. (2001) Preparation and Mechanical Properties of Polylactic Acid Composites Containing Hydroxyapatite fibers. *Biomaterials*: **22(1)**: 19-23.
85. Navarro M, Ginebra MP, Planell JA, Zeppetelli S, and Ambrosio L. (2004) Development and cell response of a new biodegradable composite scaffold for guided bone regeneration. *Journal of Materials Science: Materials in Medicine* **15(4)**: 419-422.
86. Khan YM, Katti DS, and Laurencin CT. (2004) Novel polymer-synthesized ceramic composite-based system for bone repair: an *in vitro* evaluation. *Journal of Biomedical Materials Research - Part A* **69(4)**: 728-737.
87. Rho JY, Kuhn-Spearing L, and Zioupos P (1998) Mechanical properties and the hierarchical structure of bone. *Medical Engineering & Physics* **20(2)**: 92-102.
88. Khan, Y.M., Katti, D.S., and Laurencin, C.T. (2004) Novel polymer-synthesized ceramic composite-based system for bone repair: An in vitro evaluation. *Journal of Biomedical Materials Research: A* **69**: 728-737.
89. Kikuchi M, Cho SB, Suetsugu Y, and Tanaka J. (1997) In vitro tests and in vivo tests developed TCP/CPLA composites. *Bioceramics* **10**: 407-410.
90. Du C, Cui FZ, Zhu XD, and de Groot K. (1999) Three-dimensional nano-HAP/collagen matrix loading with osteogenic cells in organ culture. *Journal of Biomedical Materials Research* **44(4)**: 407-415.
91. Webster TJ, Siegel RW, and Bizios R. (2001) Nanoceramic surface roughness enhances osteoblast and osteoclast functions for improved orthopaedic/dental implant efficacy. *Scripta Materialia* **44(8-9)**: 1639-1642.
92. Webster TJ, Ergun C, Doremus RH, Siegel RW, and Bizios R. (2000) Specific proteins mediate enhanced osteoblast adhesion on nanophase ceramics. *Journal of Biomedical Materials Research* **51(3)**: 475-483.
93. Webster TJ, Siegel RW, and Bizios R. (1999) Osteoblast adhesion on nanophase ceramics. *Biomaterials* **20(13)**: 1221-1227.
94. Dulgar Tulloch AJ, Bizios R, and Siegel RW. (2003) Nanophase alumina/poly(L-lactic acid) composite scaffolds for biomedical applications. *Materials Research Society Symposium Proceedings* **740**: 161-166.
95. Webster TJ, Siegel RW, and Bizios R. (2001) Nanoceramic surface roughness enhances osteoblast and osteoclast functions for improved orthopaedic/dental implant efficacy. *Scripta Materialia* **44(8-9)**: 1639-1642.
96. Yamasaki H and Sakai H. (1992) Osteogenic response to porous hydroxyapatite ceramics under the skin of dogs. *Biomaterials* **13(5)**: 308-312.
97. Yuan H, Kurashina K, de Bruijin JD, Li Y, de Grout K, and Zhang X. (1999) A preliminary study on osteoinduction of two kinds of calcium phosphate ceramics. *Biomaterials* **20(19)**: 1799-1806.

98. Liu H, Slamovich EB, and Webster TJ. (2005) Increased osteoblast functions on nanophase titania dispersed in poly-lactic-co-glycolic acid composites. *Nanotechnology* **16(7)**: S601-S608.
99. Webster TJ, Schadler LS, Siegel RW, and Bizios R. (2001) Mechanisms of enhanced osteoblast adhesion on nanophase alumina involve vitronectin. *Tissue Engineering* **7(3)**: 291-302.
100. Qin XY, Kim JG, and Lee JS. (1999) Synthesis and magnetic properties of nanostructured γ-Ni-Fe alloys. *Nanostructured Materials* **11(2)**: 259-270.
101. Li P, Miser DE, Rabiei S, Yadav RT, and Hajaligol MR. (2003) The removal of carbon monoxide by iron oxide nanoparticles. *Applied Catalysis B: Environmental* **43(2)**: 151-162.
102. Surowiak Z, Osinska, K, and Czekaj D. (2001) Structure and physical properties of nano-structured $Pb(Zr_{0.5}Ti_{0.5})O_3$ piezoceramics. *Proceedings of SPIE-The International Society for Optical Engineering* **4413**: 163-168.
103. Suh SW, Shin JY, Kim J, Kim J, Beak CH, Kim DI, Kim H, Jeon SS, and Choo IW. (2002) Effect of different particles on cell proliferation in polymer scaffolds using a solvent-casting and particulate leaching technique. *ASAIO Journal* **48(5)**: 460-464.
104. Shastri V P, Martin I, and Langer R. (2000) Macroporous polymer foams by hydrocarbon templating. *Proceedings of the National Academy of Sciences USA* **97**: 1970-1975.
105. Wu L, Zhang H, Zhang J, and Ding J. (2005) Fabrication of three-dimensional porous scaffolds of complicated shape for tissue engineering. I. Compression molding based on flexible-rigid combined mold. *Tissue Engineering* **11(7-8)**: 1105-1114.
106. Harris LD, Kim BS, and Mooney DJ. (1998) Open pore biodegradable matrices formed with gas foaming. *Journal of Biomedical Materials Research* **42**: 396-402.
107. Kim SS, Park MS, Jeon O, Choi CY, and Kim BS. (2006) Poly(lactide-co-lycolide)/hydroxyapatite composite scaffolds for bone tissue engineering. *Biomaterials* **27(8)**: 1399-1409.
108. Nam Y S, Yoon J J, and Park T G. (2000) A novel fabrication method of macroporous biodegradable polymer scaffolds using gas foaming salt as a porogen additive. *Journal of Biomedical Materials Research: Part B Applied Biomaterials* **53**: 1-7.
109. Whang K, Thomas C H, Healy K E, and Nuber G. (1995) Novel method to fabricate bioabsorbable scaffolds. *Polymer* **36(4)**: 837-842.
110. Liu L, Zhang, L, Ren B, Wang F, and Zhang Q. (2003) Preparation and characterization of collagen-hydroxyapatite composite used for bone tissue engineering scaffold. *Artificial Cells, Blood Substitutes, and Biotechnology* **31(4)**: 435-448.

111. Lo H, Kadiyala S, Guggino SE, and Leong KW. (1996) Poly(L-lactic acid) foams with cell seeding and controlled-release capacity. *Journal of Biomedical Materials Research* **30**: 475-484.
112. Lo H, Ponticiello MS, and Leong KW. (1995) Fabrication of controlled release biodegradable foams by phase separation. *Tissue Engineering* **1**: 15-28.
113. Schugens C, Maquet V, Grandfils C, Jerome R, and Teyssie P. (1996) Polylactide macroporous biodegradable implants for cell transplantation II. Preparation of polylactide foams for liquid-liquid phase separation. *Journal of Biomedical Materials Research* **30**: 449-461.
114. Nam YS, and Park TG. (1996) Porous biodegradable polymeric scaffolds prepared by thermally induced phase separation. *Journal of Biomedical Materials Research* **47**: 17.

Chapter 2

Nanomaterials for Better Orthopedics

Ganesan Balasundaram

1. Introduction

One of the top concerns in the design of orthopedic biomaterials is to simulate properties of bone in synthetic implant formulations. In the past, synthetic conventional materials have not served as satisfactory implants. As an example, the current average lifetime of an orthopedic implant (such as hip, knee, ankle, etc.) is only 10 to 15 years.[1-2] Clearly, such conventional materials (or those materials with constituent dimensions greater than 1 micron) have not invoked suitable cellular responses to regenerate bone to allow these devices to be successful for long periods of time. In contrast, due to their ability to mimic the dimensions of constituent components of natural bone (like proteins and hydroxyapatite), nanophase materials may be an exciting successful alternative orthopedic implant material.

The National Nanotechnology Initiative, a government initiative in the USA describes nanotechnology as: research and development aimed at understanding and working with (such as seeing, measuring and manipulating) matter at the atomic, molecular and supramolecular levels. This correlates to length scales of roughly 1 to 100 nanometres.[3] At this scale, the physical, chemical and biological properties of materials differ fundamentally and often unexpectedly from those of the corresponding bulk materials.

Due to their size, nanoscale materials often exhibit unique physical/chemical properties and can impart enhancements to engineered materials, including better magnetic properties, improved electrical and optical activity, and increased structural integrity.[4] In addition, these materials are often much more reactive than their bulk material counterparts as a result of their larger surface areas.[5]

In order to describe the promise that nanophase materials have to revolutionize orthopedic applications, this chapter will begin with the necessities to develop better implantation materials for such applications. To make the connection with nanophase materials, the chapter will then describe how nanostructured surfaces manipulate cell functions important for improving such orthopedic applications. Finally, this chapter will end with how nanophase materials can be efficiently used to fight the challenges provoked in orthopedic research. In this manner, this chapter will present a comprehensive view of how nanotechnology is being used to prevent and treat bone related problems.

2. Skeletal Complications: Osteoporosis and Bone Fracture

Osteoporosis is a disorder characterized by reduced bone strength, diminished bone density, and altered macrogeometry/microscopic architecture. The reduction in bone strength is a function of reduced bone mass and abnormal bone quality, including microscopic architecture of the bone, bone turnover, damage accumulation, and mineralization. Osteoporosis is often asymptomatic for many years until end-organ complications (fractures) occur. These fractures and their consequences, which include pain, disability, deformity, and sometimes premature death, are the only recognized clinical symptoms of osteoporosis.

To emphasize the severity of the problem, a primary goal of Healthy People 2010 is to increase the life expectancy and improve the quality of life of all individuals. The U.S. Bureau of Census has clearly demonstrated that we are an aging demographic. For example, the percentage of the population greater than 65 years of age is expected to increase from 12.4 to 23% between the years 2000 and 2100.[6] Not surprisingly, a similar upward trend is projected for the debilitating age-related disease: osteoporosis. Specifically, osteoporosis cases will rise from 10.1 million in 2002 to 13.9 million in 2020. As osteoporosis is not discriminatory, this increase is expected to occur across all racial, ethnic, and gender groups. More importantly, nationwide, approximately 1.5 million bone fractures per year are attributed to osteoporosis. Unfortunately, almost one-third of patients with hip fractures are forced to reside in nursing homes within one year of fracture and approximately 24% of hip fractures in patients aged 50 and over die in the year following the fracture.[7] Shockingly, due to the above statistics, the increase in osteoporotic fractures for the next 60 years is projected to be over 300%. The severity of this problem will be recognized nationally in a Surgeon General's Report on the "Prevention and Treatment of Osteoporosis and other Bone Disorders". For these reasons, annual direct costs for the treatment of osteoporotic fractures in the year 2003 are estimated at $17 billion in the U.S. and this number will certainly rise to staggering amounts in the years ahead.

3. Need for Better Implantation Materials for Orthopedic Application

The need for orthopedic implants is great. We currently do not have sufficient materials to treat changes in bone mass that may result from fractures, osteoporosis, and/or bone cancer. For example, orthopedic implant materials (or fixation devices) are used when changes in bone mass lead to debilitating fractures. It is the hope that these materials will repair bone non-unions quickly and effectively so that the patient can return to a normal healthy life style. Moreover, it has been speculated that the materials used today (including titanium, CoCrMo, etc.) as bone fixation devices have an overall average implant lifetime of only 10 to 15 years.[1,2] Such a limited lifetime may be appropriate for older patients who may not live past this time frame, but for an aging active baby-boomer generation, this will not suffice.

A bone implant should not only temporarily replace missing bone, but also provide a framework into which the host bone and vascular network can regenerate and heal. It should act as a scaffold to support new bone formation, blood vessels and soft tissue as they grow to connect fractured bone segments, thus strengthening the grafted area and fixating it by forming a bridge between existing bone and the graft material. However, ideally, the implant should also interact with the host tissue, recruiting and even promoting differentiation of osteogenic cells, rather than acting as a passive stage for the performance of any itinerant cells.

There are clearly two important (but not unrelated) factors for orthopedic implant material selection: the correct chemistry to support or stimulate an appropriate host response and the geometric engineering of an appropriate scaffold structure. There is a clear history of a "trial-and-error" approach for orthopedic material chemistries. While this approach has increased the lifetimes of current orthopedic implants, "trial-and-error" approaches have not overwhelmingly improved the success of bone implants.

Some of the problems continuously playing orthopedic implant failure include, but are not limited to:

- Poor initial bone growth on the surface of the implant which is to integrate, and bond into juxtaposed bone,
- Generation of wear debris in articulating components of implants that become lodged between the implant and surrounding tissue, thus leading to bone cell death, and
- Stress and strain imbalances between an implant and surrounding tissue that leads to implant loosening and eventual fracture.

To overcome many of these problems, bone implant materials need to stimulate rapid bone regeneration in order to fill in deficient bone or to fix an implant firmly within adjacent bone. Thus, to succeed as an orthopedic implant material, a material must be habitable especially for bone-forming cells (osteoblasts) such that they can colonize on the implant surface and synthesize new bone tissue. For successful implants, sufficiently regenerated bone fills the gap between an implant and juxtaposed bone, thus, the implant is attached firmly with surrounding bone.

However, this is not always the case. Frequently implant materials are not preferentially compatible with bone cells responsible for bone formation, but rather they promote the formation of undesirable soft connective tissue. Fibrous soft tissue, as opposed to hard bony tissue, has been shown to improperly fix orthopedic implants into surrounding bone which leads to loosening under physiological loading conditions and eventual implant failure.[8] Another undesired event is fibrous soft tissue formation by fibroblasts. Excessive fibrous tissue formation hinders osteoblast/osteoclast activities and, thus, less new bone regeneration between an implant and juxtaposed bone results.

The "trail-and-error" application to orthopedic implant design has not been able to develop materials that resist fibrous, soft tissue formation. Importantly, such desirable, rapid formation of new bone (not fibrous, soft tissue) will assist in decreasing the detrimental influences of wear debris generated from articulating components of orthopedic implants. For example, since full integration of an implant into surrounding bone will leave little to no room for wear debris to situate and cause bone death, proper efficient new bone formation on the surface of an implant will decrease the harmful consequences of wear debris.

As discussed, it is clear that to design better orthopedic implant materials, one needs to concentrate on cellular processes that lead to efficient new bone growth. Positive responses from osteoblasts, including increased initial adhesion, proliferation, and differentiation from non-calcium depositing to calcium depositing cells are essential. In addition, coordinated activities between osteoblasts and the bone-resorbing cells, osteoclasts, are needed to maintain healthy bone surrounding the implant. Poor communication between these cells will lead to necrotic (or dead) bone juxtaposed to the implant which is much weaker and will lead to fracture in the bone surrounding the implant. Due to the importance of these specific cellular events, the orthopedic field has turned away from "trial-and-error" engineering and is now concentrating on understanding cellular recognition of implant surfaces creating biomaterial surface properties to maximize initial cellular interactions that lead to the goal of more bone formation; such cellular events are emphasized in the next section.

3.1. Cell Recognition of Implant Surfaces

Engineers and scientists are continuously investigating novel orthopedic materials which can promote desirable responses from surrounding cells for better osseointegration. Before osteoblasts (or other cells) adhere to an implanted surface, proteins will adsorb from bodily fluids such as bone marrow, blood, and other tissues. In this manner, it has been observed that proteins initially adsorbed onto the surfaces of implants control subsequent cell adhesion.[9] Specific proteins (such as fibronectin and vitronectin) in biological fluids, such as blood plasma, mediate the adhesion, differentiation, and growth of desirable cells on an implant surface.[10-11] For this reason, many investigators are now paying close attention to manipulating initial protein adsorption events by altering select properties of implant surfaces.

Indeed, some studies have provided evidence that changes in implant surface energy, surface chemical composition, and surface features influence the type and concentration of adsorbed proteins.[12] For example, previous studies have shown that fibronectin preferentially adsorbs on calcium phosphate-coated bioactive glass compared with untreated bioactive glass and stoichiometric bioactive glass.[13] Lee and colleagues also demonstrated the control of select protein adsorption leading to greater Chinese hamster ovary cell adhesion, by oxidizing certain polymers; the same trend was also observed for fibroblasts.[14,15] Moreover, it is now well recognized that osteoblasts preferentially adhere to specific amino acid sequences such as arginine-glycine-aspartic acid (RGD) and heparin-sulfate binding regions in adsorbed proteins.[16] Accordingly, how specific amino acid sequences are exposed in adsorbed proteins to associate with binding to integrin receptors in cell membranes is critical to whether cell adhesion will occur on an implant surface.

Thus, the efficacy of bone generation is determined mainly by surface characteristics such as the chemical composition and physical properties of the implant that controls initial protein adsorption. These properties alter adsorption of proteins which mediate the adhesion of desirable (osteoblast) and undesirable (fibroblast) cells. It is believed that the lack of attention paid to understanding cellular recognition to proteins initially adsorbed on biomaterial surfaces to date is one of the key reasons why current implant do not, on average, last longer than 15 years. It is this new direction aimed at intelligently designing implant surfaces to control protein interactions important for subsequent cell adhesion that may provide answers to those problems which have plagued current orthopedic implants. Central to this approach is changing orthopedic implant chemistries and topography.

3.2. Chemistry

There have been many approaches to design next generation of improved bone implants. Representative implant materials currently being investigated include metals (CoCrMo alloys, titanium, and titanium alloys), ceramics (alumina, titania, zirconia, hydroxyapatite), polymers (polyurethane, polyethylene, and poly-lactic-co-glycolic acid [PLGA]), and biologically synthesized substances such as mineralized collagen in simulated body fluid, in which calcium and phosphate are supersaturated.[17] However, it is clear that some of these current approaches have not yet led to the design of optimal bone implant materials. For example, many metals used as orthopedic materials have shown poor osseointegration; specifically, studies have highlighted that plain (i.e., uncoated) titanium generates less bone formation to bond to surrounding bone and instead induces soft fibrous tissue formation.[18]

Conversely, in general, bioceramics have been shown to be more successful as bone replacements, either for small defects or as coatings for titanium to be used to heal large defects due to their excellent biocompatibility and interaction with bone cells. It has been demonstrated that many ceramics enhance initial adsorption of select proteins (for example, fibronectin and vitronectin) and thus, promote bone cell function that leads to osteoconductivity and osseointegration. Some studies have preadsorbed specific collagen-mimetic amino acid sequences which stimulate the specific expression of $\alpha_1\beta_1$ integrin receptors in osteoblast cell membranes to enhance alkaline phosphatase activity and matrix mineralization.[19]

Polymers have also shown some promise. For example, Underwood and colleagues demonstrated that Ca^{2+}-treated vitronectin adsorbed on polystyrene possessed a more bioactive conformation that enhanced osteoblast function compared with other materials.[20]

Collectively, these studies clearly indicate that biomaterial surface chemistry can manipulate osteoblast function. To date, changing material surface chemistry has been a primary investigative tool to enhance the performance of orthopedic implants. However, such results have not been universal and no material chemistry is the gold-standard for increasing bone regeneration; that is, in some cases it has produced better materials but in other cases it has not. Moreover it is believed that elucidation of one material property that can be used on any implant chemistry to increase bone growth may be a better approach; this is the role envisioned for nanophase materials and topography.

3.3. Topography

Another manner in which investigators have tried to improve the performance of bone implants is by manipulating surface roughness. Specially, compared with smooth surfaces, micron surface roughness (<10 μm) of titanium substrates created by sand-blasting, etching, machining and the use of micron-size metal bead coatings has enhanced osteoblast functions such as adhesion, proliferation, production of alkaline phosphatase, and deposition of calcium-containing mineral.[21-22] Many of these techniques are currently being incorporated into the orthopedic marketplace. In fact, improved osteoinduction of titanium was observed on micro porous structures compared with non-microporous titanium which did not induce bone formation at all.[23] Several studies have further suggested that other microstructural features (such as grain and particle size) promote osteoblast functions compared with smooth surfaces. In contrast to the previously mentioned method of altering biomaterial chemistry to promote bone for formation, increasing micron-surface roughness for a wide range of materials has more universally promoted bone growth. That is, this approach has proved helpful for a wide range of implant chemistries.

However, the type of roughness created in these studies (micron roughness) does not match the roughness that osteoblasts are naturally accustomed to in the body. Since bone is composed of constituent nanostructures, it is clear that instead of formulating surfaces with micron roughness, emphasis should be placed on techniques that create nanometer roughness; this is, indeed, the role nanophase materials (or materials with constituent features less than 100 nm in at least one direction) can play in universally increasing the efficacy of any orthopedic implant chemistry.

4. A New Approach: Nanophase Orthopedic Materials

While numerous advantages of nanomaterials have been elucidated for catalytic, electronic, computer, magnetic fields, few have been described for biological applications. Nanophase materials discussed in the present review are defined as materials with constituent structural units between 1-100 nm in terms of grain size if crystalline solids or particle sizes if amorphous. In fact, human bone is assembled from nanosized organic and inorganic mineral phases into large complex architectures. Specifically, calcium phosphate crystallites (200-800 Å long and 2-5 nm thick) which are similar to hydroxyapatite (HA; $Ca_{10}[PO_4][OH]_2$) compositionally and structurally are examples of naturally occurring nanomaterials.[24] In addition, other proteins in the extra cellular matrix of bone are nanostructured such as Type I collagen fibers. In this manner, by examining the fundamental structure of bone, it is clear that osteoblasts are accustomed to interacting with nanophase materials, yet the field continues to implant non-biologically inspired micron-structured materials.

This motivates the use of nanophase materials for orthopedic implants since their structure is biologically-inspired. Similar to creating micron roughness, results of bone formation on implant surfaces with nanometer roughness values seem to be universal and better than on micron roughness surfaces. In fact, when compared with conventional materials (or materials with micron grain sizes), several studies have reported improved osseointegration on nanophase surfaces created from a wide range of chemistries including ceramics, metals, polymers, and composites thereof.[11] For example, Price and colleagues showed that alumina nanometer fibers (2-4 nm > 50 nm), when consolidated, significantly stimulated osteoblast responses such as adhesion, alkaline phosphatase activity, and calcium deposition, when compared with conventional grain size alumina (Fig. 1).[25-26] Importantly, this study also demonstrated increased osteoblast function on alumina nanofibers compared with alumina nanospheres (23 nm in diameter). It was hypothesized that since alumina nanofibers are more structurally similar to that of calcium phosphate crystals and collagen fibers found in natural bone, another key parameter to emulate in nanostructures for bone replacements are there constituent fibrous nature.

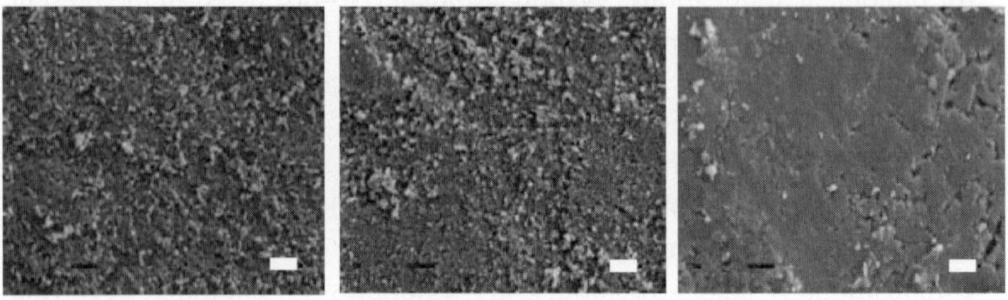

Figure 1. Representative SEM images of conventional alumina, nano-spherical alumina and alumina nanofibers. Bone cell functions are enhanced on nanofiber alumina compared with nanospherical alumina. Bone cell functions are enhanced on nano-spherical alumina compared with conventional alumina. Bars = 1 μm. Adapted from[25].

The importance of nanofibers for bone regeneration has been demonstrated in other studies. Specifically, greater in vitro osteoblast adhesion has been observed on helical rosette nanotube-coated titanium compared with uncoated titanium (Fig. 2). Helical rosette nanotubes are novel organic nanotube formulations that mimic the dimensions of the nanostructure of bone components.[27] In this manner, this study demonstrated that traditional, currently-used, titanium implants can be transformed into bioactive formulations through the use of nanostructure coatings like helical rosette nanotubes.

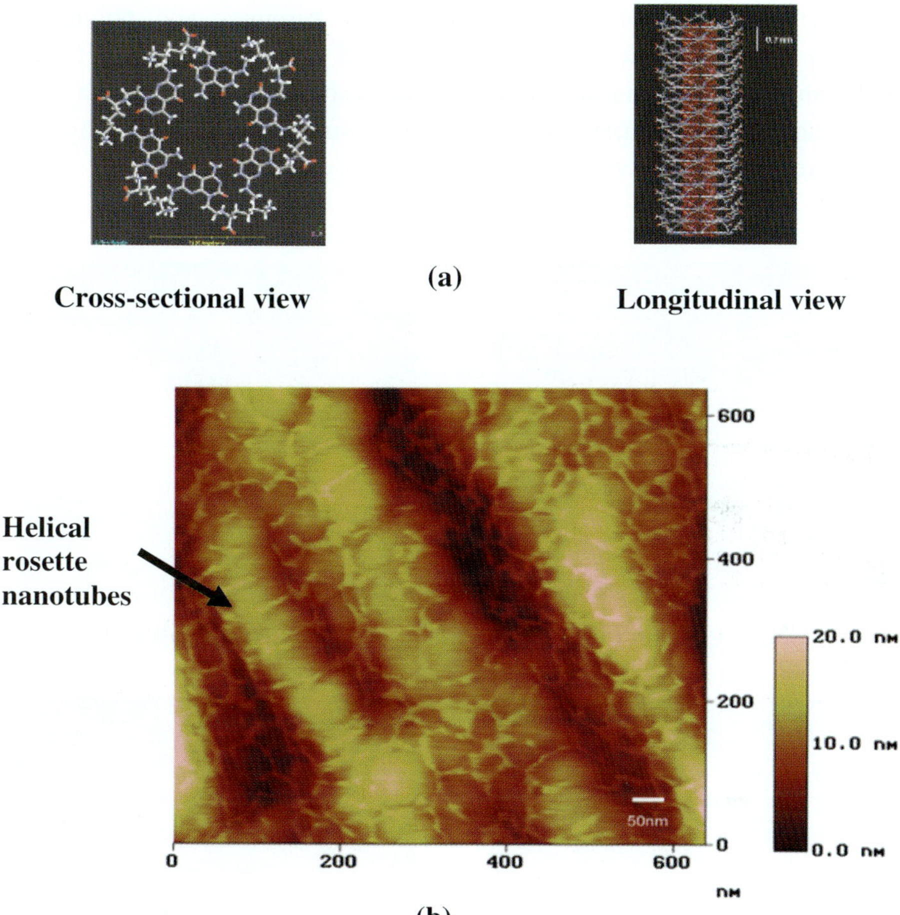

Figure 2. Helical rosette nanotubes. Drawing of the cross-sectional (left) and longitudinal (right) view of self-assembled helical rosette nanotubes is depicted in (a) while helical rosette nanotubes coated on titanium is depicted in (b). Note the nanophase dimensions of these organic tubes. Increased osteoblast functions have been observed on helical rosette nanotubes coated on titanium. Adapted from[27].

Other novel nanostructures that have increased responses from osteoblasts leading to more efficient deposition of calcium-containing mineral include: nanometals (Fig. 3), carbon nanofibers/nanotubes

(Fig. 4), nanopolymers, nanocomposites of ceramics and polymers (Fig. 5).[28-30] This new evidence of increased osteoblast function for a wide range of nanomaterial chemistries suggests that such trends may be independent of the underlying material chemistry and dependent only on the degree of nanostructured surface roughness created.

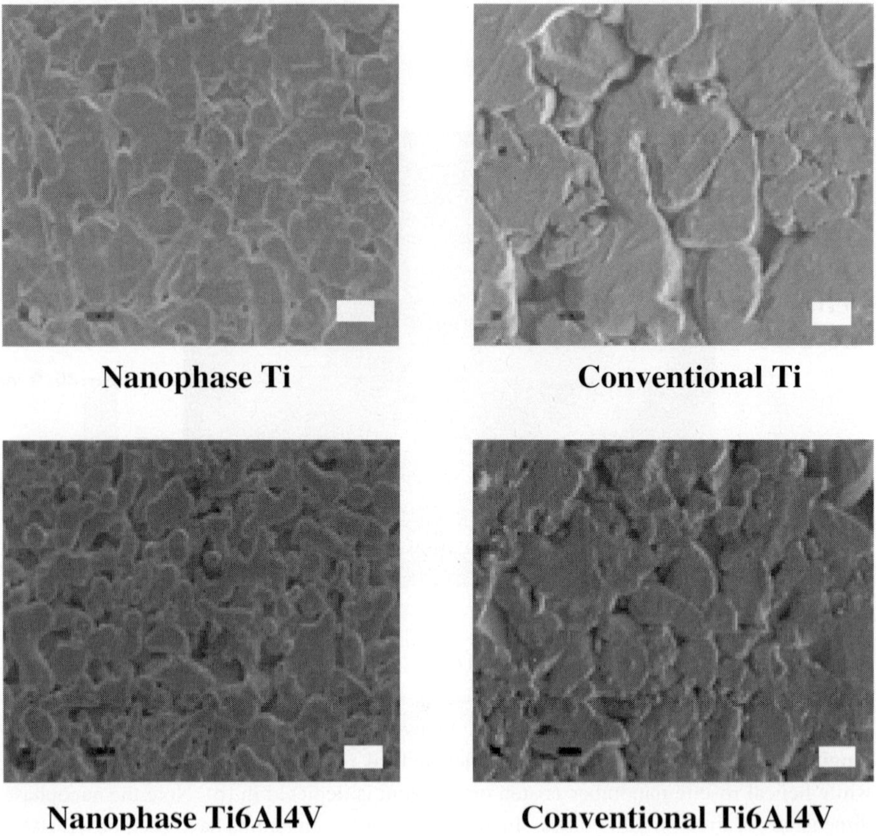

Figure 3. SEM images depicting conventional titanium in comparison with nanophase titanium (Ti) and conventional Ti6Al4V in comparison with nanophase Ti6Al4V. Bars represent 10 μm for conventional and 1 μm for nanophase metals, respectively. Bone cell functions are enhanced on nanophase compared with conventional metals. Adapted from[28].

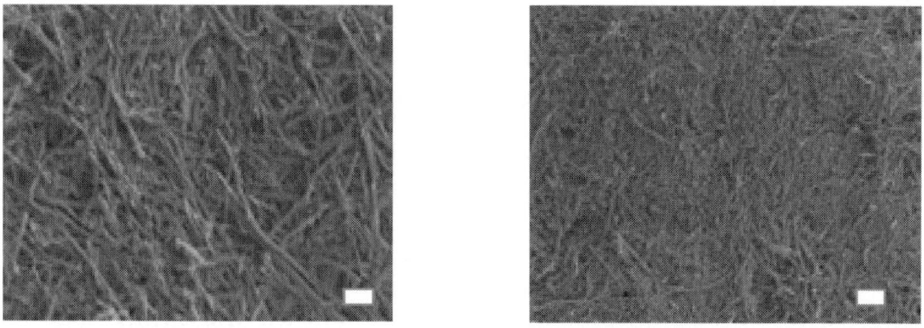

Conventional carbon fiber compacts **Nanophase carbon fiber compacts**

Figure 4. SEM images depicting conventional carbon fibers (0.125 mm diameter) in comparison with nanophase carbon fibers (60 nm diameter). Bars represent 1 μm. Bone cell functions are enhanced on nanophase compared with conventional carbon fibers. Adapted from [29].

PLGA: Conventional TiO_2 (70:30 wt.%)

Nanophase TiO_2

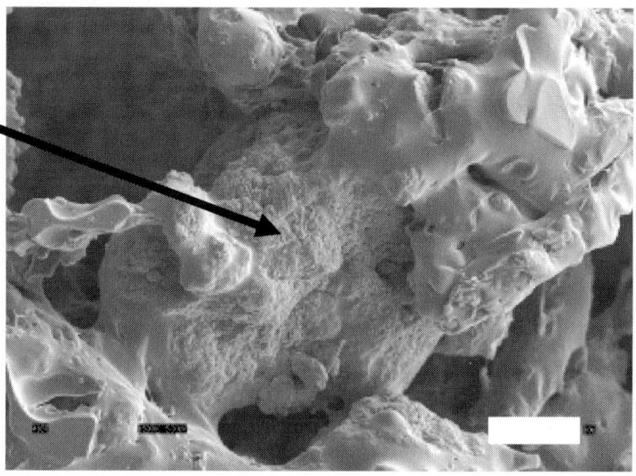

PLGA: Nanophase TiO_2 (70:30 wt.%)

Figure 5. SEM images depicting PLGA composites containing conventional titania (4.120 mm grain size) in comparison with nanophase titania (32 nm grain size). Weight percentage: 70/30 PLGA/titania. Bars represent 10 μm. Bone cell functions are enhanced on polymer composites containing nanophase compared with conventional ceramics. PLGA: poly-lactic-co-glycolic acid. Adapted from[29].

In the following sections, material property benefits of nanophase materials that may be accounting for such trends of increased bone cell functions pertinent to orthopedic applications are expanded.

4.1. Benefits of Nanophase Bone Implant Materials

As mentioned, optimal surface properties are desired to promote new bone growth. Since surface properties vary with the grain size of a material, there is excitement concerning the use of nanomaterials in orthopedics, especially when considering that they can be manufactured to stimulate the size of constituent components of bone. Due to the importance of initial protein interactions with implant surfaces, it is clear that if surface properties are changed, cell functions will be influenced. In this regard, it is thought that nanoscale materials can interact with select proteins more effectively than conventional materials to mediate osteoblast functions.

Recent studies have indeed demonstrated that the adsorption and conformation (or bioactivity) of proteins that mediate specific osteoblast adhesion (such as fibronectin and vitronectin) are enhanced on nanophase materials.[12,31] Specifically, Woo and colleagues reported that three dimensional nanofibrous scaffolds selectively adsorbed more proteins, including fibronectin and vitronectin, compared with a solid pore wall consisting of the same material: poly (L-lactic acid).[32] This led to increased osteoblast functions on nanofibrous polymer scaffolds. One of the main reasons why nanophase materials attract select proteins to their surface is due to their altered surface energetics compared with conventional materials (>100 nm).

Moreover, studies have highlighted altered protein bioactivity when adsorbed to nanophase compared with conventional materials.[11-12] Specifically, the peptide sequence, RGD, was more exposed when vitronectin was adsorbed to nanophase compared with conventional ceramics. It is thought that the bioactivity of select proteins is altered on nanophase materials due to both greater wettability and surface features closer to the size of protein itself (the nanoscale); these novel properties of nanophase materials are expanded in the proceeding section.

4.2. Wettability

A number of surface properties are changed when grain size is reduced into the nanometer regimen. Specifically, Wen and colleagues measured grain boundary volume percentage with grain sizes ranging from 2 μm to 2 nm (Table 1).[33] As expected, they found greater numbers of grain boundaries at the surface of nanophase compared with conventional materials. In addition, compared with larger grain counterparts, nanophase materials possessed higher surface area and altered electron distributions.[34] Collectively, since proteins are charged molecules, such properties will change surface energetics to influence protein interactions that mediate cell adhesion.

Table 1. Grain boundary volume percentage for conventional and nanophase materials. Adapted from [33].

Materials	Conventional	Nanophase			
Grain Size (nm)	2000	20	10	4	2
Grain Boundary thickness (nm)	0.6	0.6	0.6	0.6	0.6
Grain Boundaray volume %	0.09	9.0	18.0	42.6	80.5

For example, Webster and colleagues demonstrated that aqueous contact angles were three times smaller when alumina grain size was decreased from 167 to 24 nm.[12] They also reported that the adsorption of vitronectin, which stimulates osteoblast adhesion, increased on nanophase ceramics with greater wettability.[35] Moreover, when vitronectin adsorbed on nanophase ceramics, it was unfolded to a larger extent that on conventional ceramics which exposed larger numbers of osteoblast adhesive epitopes in the absorbed proteins. Similar increased unfolding and exposure of osteoblast adhesive epitopes was demonstrated for fibronectin on nanophase ceramics, another key protein for encouraging osteoblast function.[36]

Similar to single-phase ceramics, increased wettability of polymer composites have been achieved through the use of nanophase ceramics in order to increase bone cell function. Specifically, Kay and colleagues demonstrated that titania nanosized particles embedded in PLGA promoted osteoblast adhesion compared with conventional sized titania (> 100 nm) in PLGA.[37] PLGA containing nanoparticles of titania were more hydrophilic than those containing conventional titania. Lastly, this same trend of enhancing osteoblast function by creating more wettable surfaces through the use of nanophase materials holds for metals as well. For example, osteoblast deposited more calcium on hydrophilic metal surfaces composed separately of nanometer compared with conventional Ti, Ti6Al4V, and CoCrMo. Interestingly, osteoblasts preferentially adhered at metal particle boundaries when metal nanograin sizes were less than 1 μm.[28] Although not tested to date, the authors speculate that either vitronectin or fibronectin may be adsorbing specifically at metal nanoparticles boundaries and, thus, are initiating osteoblast attachment at those sites.

4.3. Surface Roughness

As mentioned, surface roughness is a crucial property influencing cell response. Clearly, nanophase materials exhibit different scales of surface roughness compared with conventional surfaces. One of the clearest studies highlighting the importance of nanometer roughness was conducted by Price and colleagues.[38] In this study, polymer casts of consolidated carbon nanofiber-based materials were created, which had previously been shown to promote bone cell function compared with consolidated conventional dimensioned carbon fiber materials. Importantly, the study demonstrated increased osteoblast adhesion on polymer casts of nanophase carbon fibers compared with polymer of the conventional carbon fibers; the same trend observed for nanophase compared with conventional carbon fibers. In this manner, the nanometer topography as well as the subsequent ability to enhance osteoblast function on the carbon nanofiber substrates was transferred to a completely different chemistry. Polymer casts of composites of polycarbonate urethane/carbon nanotubes also promoted osteoblast function compared with casts of polycarbonate urethane/conventional carbon tubes.[39]

In addition, the importance of a nanometer roughness on bone cell function has been shown by creating ceramic substrates of the same crystallinity, crystal phase, and chemistry, altering only in degree of nanometer surface features. This was carried by Webster and colleagues for nanophase compared with conventional alumina, titania, and hydroxyapatite.[11] Nanophase roughness on these nanophase ceramics improved both osteoblastic and osteoclastic responses, whilst simultaneously inhibiting fibroblast function. For instance, greater osteoblast deposition of calcium containing mineral and the number of resorption pits created by osteoclasts correlated with increased nanometer surface roughness ranging from 17 to 20 nm for alumina.[40] Supporting evidence of decreased fibroblast function on nanophase ceramics has been presented by Mustafa and colleagues who suggested that ceramics with increasing surface roughness (from 60 nm to 300 nm) decreased initial fibroblast adhesion compared with smooth surfaces.[41] Similar trends have been reported for PLGA of the same surface chemistry but altering only in degree of nanometer surface roughness (50-100 nm).[42] Specifically, Washburn and colleagues demonstrated that osteoblastic cells reduced proliferation and possibly increased differentiation into calcium-depositing cells on polymer nanotopographies grater than 1.1 nm.[43]

Lastly, studies by Dalby and colleagues have also indicated the importance of nanometer surface structures (without altering material chemistry) in controlling cell functions. Specifically, they reported that islands of 95 nm in height decreased fibroblast proliferation compared with those of 13 nm in height on a copolymer mixture of polystyrene and polybromostyrene.[44] Although not measured, decreased sub-confluent fibroblast proliferation could mean decreased differentiation and synthesis of undesirable fibrous tissue. In a subsequent study, the authors suggested that fibroblast changed their cytoskeleton arrangements on the polymer islands in the nanometer regime which suppressed spreading and formation of confluent cell layers.[45] Another study has suggested that smooth muscle cell numbers were greater on nanometer compared with conventional roughness values, thus, adding validity that nanometer surface features may influence a wide range of cell functions yet largely not studied to date.[46]

Collectively, these studies imply that cell responses might be more sensitive to changes in surface roughness in the nanometer (<100 nm) compared with conventional (>100 μm) regimes and sensitivity may vary with cell type. Most importantly, for orthopedic implant applications, the news is very positive, indicating increased osteoblast and osteoclast activity, while at the same time decreased fibroblast function on materials with nanostructured features which may lead to improve osseointegrative potentials.

5. Influence of Nanomaterials Functionalized with Cell Adhesive Peptides on Osteoblast Functions

Another popular method that has been used to improve orthopedic implant performance involves functionalizing the aforementioned nanomaterials with cell adhesive peptides. Specifically, since the identification of the RGD sequence in mediating the attachment of cells through specific ligand-receptor interactions, researchers have been depositing RGD-containing peptides on to biomaterials to promote cell attachment.[47-49] In order to derivatize the peptide molecules in a stable manner to the surfaces, covalent immobilization of the active peptide is necessary.[50] The use of covalently coupled small peptides allows some control over the density and orientation of ligand attachment. For the peptide functionalization of nanomaterials, several approaches have been explored on nano materials and currently the use of maleimide chemistry is favored.[51] The maleimide-terminated surfaces are then coupled with a peptide through the thiol group on the terminal cysteine of the peptide. The maleimide groups react efficiently with thiol-terminated ligands. It is important to note that although aminophase chemistry has been used for glass, only a few reports exist in the literature for its use on nanophase materials (particularly, nano-hydroxyapatite particles).

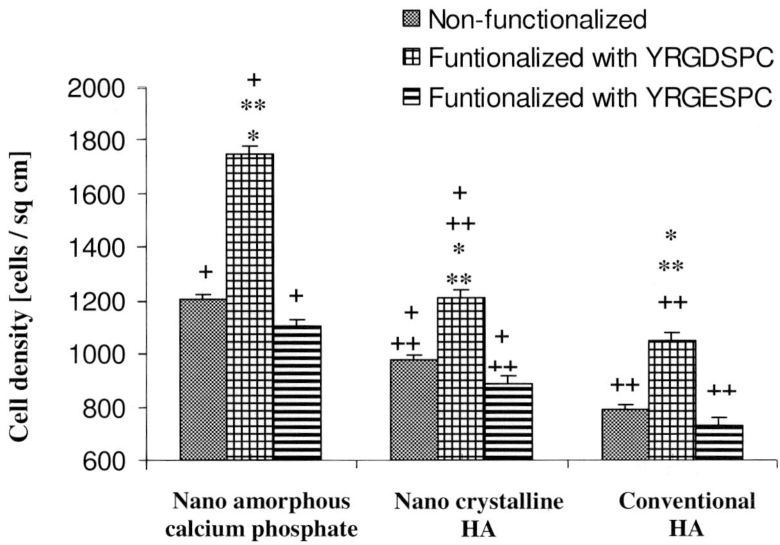

Figure 6. Greatest osteoblast adhesion on nano-amorphous calcium phosphate compacts functionalized with YRGDSPC. (a) nano-amorphous calcium phosphate, (b) nano-crystalline hydroxyapatite, and (c) conventional hydroxyapatite. Values are mean ± SEM; n=3; *p<0.01 compared to respective non-functionalized compacts, **p<0.01 compared to respective compacts functionalized with YRGESPC (negative control), +p<0.01 compared to respective conventional HA functionalization, and ++p<0.01 compared to respective nano amorphous calcium phosphate functionalization. Adapted from[51].

Our recent study provided the information that nanometer crystalline hydroxyapatite (HA) and amorphous calcium phosphate compacts could be chemically functionalized with the arginine-glycine-aspartic acid (RGD) peptide sequence using aforementioned maleimide chemistry.[51] Crystalline HA and amorphous calcium phosphate nanoparticles were synthesized by a wet chemical process followed by a hydrothermal treatment for 2 hours at 200°C and 70°C, respectively. Results showed that the immobilization of the cell adhesive RGD sequence increased osteoblast adhesion compared to those non-functionalized and those functionalized with the non cell adhesive control peptide (RGE) after 4 hours (Fig. 6). However, surprisingly, results also showed that the adhesion of osteoblasts on non-functionalized amorphous nanoparticulate calcium phosphate was similar to conventional HA functionalized with

RGD. Osteoblast adhesion on nanocrystalline HA (unfunctionalized and functionalized with RGD) was below that of the respective functionalized amorphous calcium phosphate but above that of the respective functionalized conventional HA. Further, this study suggested that decreasing the particulate size into the nanometer regime and reducing crystallinity of calcium phosphate based materials may promote osteoblast adhesion to the same degree as the well-established techniques of functionalizing conventional HA with RGD. In this manner, results from this study suggested that both nano amorphous calcium phosphate and nano crystalline HA should be further studied for applications that necessitate bone growth.

6. Future Challenges

Although nanostructured implant materials may have many potential advantages in the context of promoting bone cell responses, it is important to remember that studies on nanophase materials have only just begun; there are still many other issues regarding health that must be answered. Most importantly, influences of nanoparticulates on human health are not well understood, whether exposure occurs through the manufacturing of nanophase materials or through the implantation of nanophase materials. Clearly, detailed studies in this context are required if nanoparticles are to be used in these systems.[52]

Nanoparticles may also become loose through the degradation of implanted polymeric materials through oxidation and/or hydrolysis which accelerates exposure of materials. Corrosion of metals once implanted can also cause release of nanoparticulates and, thus, contribute toxicity to biological environments. Oxidation accelerates the degradation of metals and the release of metal ions such as Al^{3+}, Ni^{2+}, Cr^{6+}, Co^{2+}. Savarino and colleagues demonstrated that high concentrations of Cr^{6+} decreased white blood cell numbers and caused toxic effects in lymphatic organs.[53]

In addition, nanoparticles can be generated at artificial joints where friction between two surfaces is high. The outcome of micron-sized wear debris on bone health has been well-studied for several decades.

For instance, ultra high-molecular-weight polyethylene often used as acetabular cups become brittle through oxidation and, thus, become susceptible to wear. Conventional size wear debris (i.e., micron) triggers osteolysis as well as further wearing (third-body wear).[54-56]

In contrast, the influence of nanoparticulate wear debris (or particles in general) on bone cell health is only just beginning to be understood. It has been speculated that the effects of nanotubes on lungs are more toxic than quartz dust. One study showed that nanometer titania particles (50 nm) and carbon nanotubes (20 × 100 nm) induced morphological changes in neutrophils and decreased the overall cell survival rate.[57]

On the contrary, other studies have demonstrated increased cell viability in the presence nanometer, compared with conventional particles.[20] Specifically, nanophase materials did not stimulate cytotoxicity but even redeemed the toxic effects observed on osteoblast viability in the presence of conventionally sized particles. In this study, osteoblast proliferation was not negatively influenced by alumina and titania nanoparticles whereas conventional particles of the same chemistry and crystalline phase increased cell death and slowed cell proliferation. The potential lack of nanoparticle toxicity was also demonstrated on coatings of pigment-grade titania particles as nanorods and nanodots of titania (<50 nm) which did not result in as much lung inflammation when compared with larger particle sizes (>300 nm).[58]

Obviously, further tests and studies concerning the toxicity of nanophase materials need to be conducted and expanded before the benefits of nanotechnology in orthopedic applications can be realized. However, it is important to emphasize that such studies need accurate comparisons when determining health influences of nanometer compared with conventionally-sized particles of the same size and crystallinity.

In summary, despite the challenges that lie ahead, significant evidence now exists elucidating that nanophase materials represent an important growing area of research that may improve bonding between an implant and surrounding bone. Even if nanophase materials do not provide the ultimate answer for increasing bone cell responses, we have learned a tremendous amount of information concerning bone cell recognition with nanostructured surfaces that will most certainly aid in improving orthopedic implant efficacy.

Bibliography

1. Palin E, Liu H, Webster TJ. (2005) Increased osteoblast adhesion on polymer casts of nanostructured ceramics. *Nanotechnology* **16**: 1828-1836.
2. Emery DFG, Clarke HJ, Grover ML. (1997), Stanmore total hip replacement in younger patients: review of a group of patients under 50 years of age at operation. *Journal of Bone and Joint Surgery* **79**: 240-246.
3. Scott NR. (2005) State of the art *Rev. Sci. Tech. Off. Int. Epiz.*: **24**: 425-434.
4. Thomas K. (2005) Possibilities of nano. *Toxicological Sci.* **87**:316-320.
5. Murray CB, Kagan CR, Bawendi MG (2000) Advances in technology. *Science*: **287**: 1989-1994.
6. Palin, E, Liu H, Webster TJ. (2005) Increased osteoblast adhesion on polymer casts of nanostructured ceramics. *Nanotechnology* **16**: 1828-1836.
7. http://www.nof.org/osteoporosis/diseasefacts.htm
8. Anderson JM, Gristine AG, Hanson SR. (1996) Cell interactions with materials. In: *Biomaterial Science* Ratner BD, Hoffman AS, Schoen FJ, Lemons JE (eds.), Academic Press, Inc., San Deigo, pp. 165-214.
9. Schakenraad JM, Biomaterials. In: *Biomaterial Science*, Ratner BD, Hoffman AS, Schoen FJ, Lemons JE (eds.), Academic Press, Inc., San Deigo, pp. 140-141.
10. Dee KC, Puleo DA, Bizios R. (2002) Biomaterials. In: *An Introduction to Tissue-Biomaterial Interactions*, Dee KC, Puleo DA, Bizios R (eds.), John Wiley & Sons, Inc., Hoboken, New Jersey, pp. 37-52.
11. Webster TJ. (2003) Nanotechnology for the next generation of orthopedic implants. In: *Advances in Chemical Engineering*, Ying J (ed), Academic Press Inc., CA, pp. 125-166.
12. Webster TJ, Ergun C, Doremus RH, Siegel RW, Bizios R. (2000) Enhanced osteoblast functions on nanophase ceramics. *J. Biomed. Mater. Res.* **51**: 475-479.
13. El-Ghannam A, Ducheyne P, Shapiro IM. (1999) Effect of serum proteins on osteoblast adhesion to surface-modified bioactive glass and hydroxyapatite. *J. Orthop. Res.* **17**: 340-345.
14. Lee JH, Lee HB. (1993) Improved bioceramics. *J. Biomater. Sci. Polym.* **4**: 467-475.
15. Ruardy TG, Schakenraad JM, van der Mei HC, Busscher HJ. (1995) Adhesion and spreading of human skin fibroblasts on physicochemically characterized gradient surfaces. *J. Biomed. Mater. Res.* **29**: 1415-1423.
16. Ruoslahti E. (1994) RGD and other recognition sequences for integrins. *Annu. Rev. Cell. Dev. Biol.* **12**:697-715.
17. Mequita P, Branco R, Afonso A, Vasconcelos M, Cavalheiro J. (2004) Mineralized membranes for. bone regeneration. *J. Biomed. Mater. Res.* **254**: 1091-1094.

18. Soballe K, Overgaard S, Hansen ES, Brokstedt-Rasmussen H, Lind M, Bunger C. (1999) A review of ceramic coatings for implant fixation. *J. Long Term Eff. Med. Implants* **9**: 131-151.
19. Reyes CD, Garcia AJ. (2004) Alpha2beta1 integrin-specific collagen-mimetic surfaces supporting osteoblastic differentiation. *J. Biomed. Mater. Res. A.*, **69**: 591-600.
20. Underwood PA, Steele JG, Dalton BA. (1993) Effects of polystyrene surface chemistry on the biological activity of solid phase fibronectin and vitronectin, analysed with monoclonal antibodies. *J. Cell. Sci.* **104**: 793-803.
21. Anselme K, Bigerelle M, Noel B, Iost A, Hardouin P. (2002) Effect of grooved titanium substratum on human osteoblastic cell growth. *J. Biomed. Mater. Res.* **60**: 529-540.
22. Boyan BD, Lohmann CH, Sisk M, Liu Y, Sylvia VL, Cochran D L, Dean DD, Schwartz Z. (2001) Both cyclooxygenase-1 and cyclooxygenase-2 mediate osteoblast response to titanium surface roughness. *J. Biomed. Mater. Res.* **55**: 350-359.
23. Fujibayashi S, Neo M, Kim H, Kobuko T, Nakamura T. (2004) Osteoinduction of porous bioactive titanium metal. *Key. Eng. Mater.* **254**: 443-450.
24. Cowin CG. (1987) Biomaterials. In: *Handbook of Bioengineering* Skalak R, Chien, R (eds), McGraw Hill, New York.
25. Price RL, Gutwein LG, Kaledin L, Tepper F, Webster TJ. (2003) Nanometer surface roughness increases select osteoblast adhesion on carbon nanofiber compacts. *J. Biomed. Mater. Res. A.* **67**: 1284-1294.
26. Webster TJ, Ergun C, Doremus RH, Siegel RW, Bizios R. (2000) Specific osteoblast adhesion on nanophase ceramics. *Biomaterials* **21**: 1803-1809.
27. Chun AL, Moralez JG, Webster TJ, Fenniri H. (2005) Helical rosette nanotubes: a biomimetic coating for orthopedics? *Biomaterials* **26**: 7304-7309.
28. Webster TJ, Ejiofor JU. (2004) Increased osteoblast adhesion on nanostructured metals. *Biomaterials* **19**: 4731-4739.
29. Webster TJ, Smith TA. (2005) Greater osteoblast functions on nanoceramic polymer composites. *J. Biomed. Mater. Res. A.* **74**: 677-688.
30. Kay S, Thapa A, Webster TJ. (2002) Increased chondrocyte and osteoblast functions on nanoceramic polymer composites. *Tissue. Eng.* **5**: 753-760.
31. Webster TJ, Siegel RW, Bizios R. (2000) Increased osteoblast adhesion on nanophase ceramics. *Biomaterials* **20**: 1221-1225.
32. Woo KM, Chen VJ, Ma PX. (2003) Nano-fibrous scaffolding architecture selectively enhances protein adsorption contributing to cell attachment. *J. Biomed. Mater. Res. A.* **67**: 531-540.
33. Wen S, Yan D. (1995) Grain boundary in some nanomaterials. *Ceramics Inter.* **2**: 109-115.
34. Klabunde K J, Stark J, Koper O. (1996) Nanocrystals as stoichiometric reagents with unique surface chemistry. *J. Phys. Chem.* **100**: 121-125.

35. Thomas CH, McFarland CD, Jenkins MJ, Rezania A, Steele JG, Healy KE. (1997) The role of vitronectin in the attachment and spatial distribution of bone-derived cells on materials with patterned surface chemistry. *J. Biomed. Mater. Res.* **37**: 81-93.
36. Webster TJ, Ergun C, Doremus R H, Siegel RW, Bizios R. (2001) Specific proteins mediate cell adhesion on nanophase ceramics. *Biomaterials* **22**: 1327-1338.
37. Kay S, Thapa A, Haberstroh K.M, Webster TJ. (2002) Greater chondrocyte functions of nanophase ceramic composites. *Tissue. Eng.* **8**: 753-759.
38. Price RL, Ellison K, Haberstroh KM, Webster TJ. (2004) Selective osteoblast adhesion on carbon nanofibers. *J. Biomed. Mater. Res.* **70**: 129-135.
39. Webster TJ, Waid MC, McKenzie JL, Price RL, Ejiofor JU. (2004) Carbon nanofibers/nanotubes for neural and orthopedic applications. *Nanotechnology*, **15**: 48-54.
40. Webster TJ, Seigel RW, Bizios R. (2001) Nanophase materials for orthopedic applications. *Scripta. Mater.* **44**: 1639-1645.
41. Mustafa K, Oden A, Wennerberg A, Hultenby K, Arvidson K. (2005) The influence of surface topography of ceramic abutments on the attachment and proliferation of human oral fibroblasts. *Biomaterials* **26**: 373-379.
42. Vance RJ, Miller DC, Thapa A, Haberstroh KM, Webster TJ. (2004) Decreased fibroblast functions on nanostructured polymers. *Biomaterials* **25**: 2095-2100.
43. Washburn NR, Yamada KM, Imon Jr, CG, Kennedy SB, Amis EJ. (2004) High-throughput investigation of osteoblast response to polymer crystallinity: influence of nanometer-scale roughness on proliferation. *Biomaterials* **25**: 1215-1223.
44. Dalby MJ, Riehle MO, Johnstone J, Affrossman S, Curtis AS. (2002) In vitro reaction of endothelial cells to polymer demixed nanotopography. *Biomaterials* **23**: 2945-2955.
45. Dalby MJ, Riehle MO, Johnstone H, Affrossman S, Curtis AS. (2003) Fibroblast reaction to island topography: changes in cytoskeleton and morphology with time. *Biomaterials* **24**: 927-935.
46. Thapa A, Webster TJ, Haberstroh KM. (2003) Increased bladder smooth muscle cell functions on nanostructured plymers. *J. Biomed. Mater. Res. A* **67**: 1374-1381.
47. Durrieu MC, Pallu S, Guillemot F, Bareille R, Amedee J, Baquey CH, Labrugere C, Dard M. (2004) Grafting RGD containing peptides onto hydroxyapatite to promote osteoblastic cells adhesion. *J. Mater. Sci. Mater. Med.* **15**: 779-786.
48. Porte-Durrieu MC, Guillemot F, Pallu S, Labrugere C, Brouillaud B, Bareille R, Amedee J, Barthe N, Dard M, Baquey CH. (2004) Influence of roughness on cell responses. *Biomaterials* **25**: 4837-4841.
49. Porte-Durrieu MC, Labrugere C, Villars F, Lefebvre F, Dutoya S, Guette A, Bordenave L, Baquey C. (2003) Influence of roughness on cell responses. *J. Biomed. Mater. Res.*, 46, pp. 368.

50. Danczyk RB, Krieder A, Webster TJ, HogenEsch H, Rundell A. (2003) Comparison of antibody functionality using different immobilization methods. *Biotechnology and Bioengineering* **84**: 215-220.
51. Balasundaram G, Sato M, Webster T.J. (2006) Using hydroxyapatite nanoparticles and decreased crystallinity to promote osteoblast adhesion similar to functionalizing with RGD. *Biomaterials* **14**: 2798-2804.
52. Sun ZL, Wataha, JC, Hanks CT. (1997) Effects of metal ions on osteoblast-like cell metabolism and differentiation. *J. Biomed. Mater. Res.* **34**: 29-35.
53. Savarino L, Granchi D, Ciapetti G, Stea S, .Donati DE, Zinghi G, Fontanesi G, Rotini R, Montanaro L. (1999) Effects of metal ions on white blood cells of patients with failed total joint arthroplasties *J. Biomed. Mater. Res.* **47**: 543-555.
54. Fisher J, McEwen HM, Tipper JL, Galvin AL, Ingram J, Kamali A, Stone MH, Ingham E. (2004) Wear, debris, and biologic activity of cross-linked polyethylene in the knee: benefits and potential concerns. *Clin. Orthop. Relat. Res.* **428**: 114-128.
55. Green TR, Fisher J, Stone M, Wroblewski BM, Ingham E. (1998) Polyethylene particles of a 'critical size' are necessary for the induction of cytokines by macrophages in vitro. *Biomaterials* **19**: 2297.
56. Que Q, Topoleski LD. (2000) Third-body wear of cobalt-chromium-molybdenum implant alloys initiated by bone and poly(methyl methacrylate) particles. *J. Biomed. Mater. Res.* **50**: 322-330.
57. Tamura K, Takashi N, Akasaka T. (2004) Histomorphometric evidence for osteoclast-mediated bone resorption in metastatic breast cancer.*Key. Engr. Mater.* **254**: 919.
58. Warheit DB. (2004). Nanoparticles: health impact? *Materials Today* **32**: 35-40.

Chapter 3

Anodization: A Promising Nano-modification Technique for Titanium for Orthopedic Applications

Chang Yao and Thomas J. Webster

1. Introduction

As one of the valve metals (including Ti, Al, Ta, Nb, V, Hf, W), titanium is protected by a thin titanium oxide layer which spontaneously forms on its surface when exposed to air or other oxygen containing environments. This oxide passive layer is typically 2 to 5 nm thick and is responsible for the well-documented corrosion resistance property of titanium and its alloys.[1] Because of this and their excellent mechanical properties, titanium and its alloys are widely used in orthopedic and dental applications. However, the native TiO_2 layer is not bioactive enough to form a direct bonding with bone, which means the lack of osseointegration to juxtaposed bone might lead to long term failure after implantation.[2] Specifically, the 10 to 15 year lifetime of current titanium-based orthopedic implants is not as long as expected by many patients.[3]

As a result, many attempts have been made to improve the surface properties of titanium-based implants (e.g., topography, chemistry and surface energy), which directly determine the implant-environment interactions after implantation. These surface modification techniques include mechanical methods (e.g., sand-blasting), chemical methods (e.g. acid etching), coatings (e.g., plasma spraying), etc.[4-9] Through these conventional approaches, a better bonding ability with bone has been achieved due to the creation of a optimum micro-scale surface roughness, a more favorable surface chemistry, and/or a new morphology preferred by bone-forming cells (or osteoblasts). However, neither these mechanical nor chemical methods have the ability to produce controlled surface topographies. Moreover, these methods have the potential to form surface residuals. Thus, alternative methods to modify titanium surfaces are highly desirable for promoting new bone growth.

Other attempts to improve bone-bonding involves coating titanium-based implants with hydroxyapatite (HA) or other calcium phosphates, which is commonly accomplished by plasma spraying.[2] This is based on the fact that HA and other calcium phosphates are the main inorganic components of bone and they have been shown by many to directly bond to juxtaposed bone.[10-13] Unfortunately, such coatings have long-term failures due to weak adhesion to the metal substrate and dissolution once implanted. Therefore, an alternative method to deposit HA firmly onto titanium surfaces with optimal bioactivity is highly desirable for orthopedic applications.

In this light, a current strategy is to modify titanium-based implants to possess nanometer surface features considering that natural bone is a nanostructured material. It is important to note that type I collagen (organic matrix of bone) is a triple helix 300 nm in length, 0.5 nm in width, and periodicity of 67 nm while HA (inorganic mineral phase of bone) are approximately 20 to 40 nm long. Besides, HA crystals are uniquely patterned within the collagen network.[14] These indicate that bone cells may be used to an environment in nano-scale rather than micro-scale. Recently, human osteoblasts were observed to initially adhere to grain boundaries on both nanophase and conventional titanium; greater osteoblast adhesion was found on nanophase titanium that possessed more grain boundaries on the surface.[15] However, the mechanical strength of this nanophase titanium (compacts of nanoparticles) was not high enough for use as a bulk material like titanium alloys through metallurgy techniques. Proper nanometer surface modification methods for current titanium-based implants are, thus, being actively pursued.

An electrochemical method known as anodization or anodic oxidation is a well-established surface modification technique for valve metals to produce protective layers.[4] It has been successfully used as a surface treatment for orthopedic implants in the past few decades and it has some new advances recently. This chapter will present an overview of anodization and discuss processing parameters, microstructure and composition, biological responses of anodized titanium which are pertinent for orthopedic applications. Finally, this chapter will also discuss mechanisms of enhanced osteoblast functions on anodized titanium that possesses nanometer structures.

2. Anodization of Titanium

2.1. Basics of Anodization Process

Typical anodization procedures include alkaline cleaning, acid activation, and electrolyte anodizing. Acid activation is performed in a mixture of nitric acid and hydrofluoric acid (HF) to remove the natural titanium oxide layer and surface contaminants. The electrolyte anodization is carried out in an electrochemical cell which usually has a three-electrode configuration (titanium anode, platinum cathode and Ag/AgCl reference electrode). When a constant voltage or current is applied between the anode and cathode, electrode reactions (oxidation and reduction) in combination of field-driven ion diffusion (Fig. 1) lead to the formation of an oxide layer on the anode surface.

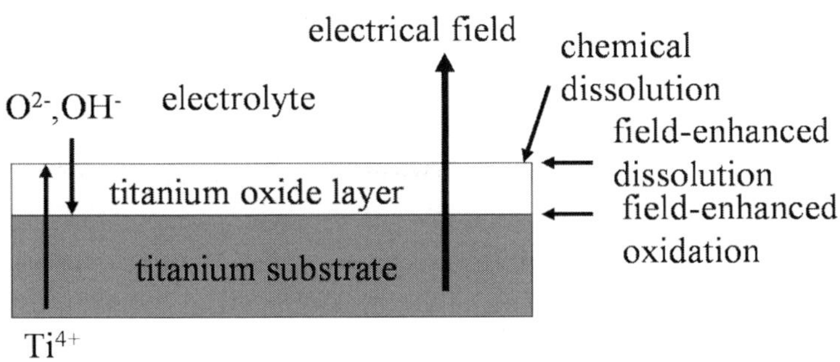

Figure 1. Schematics of ion diffusion under an electric field during anodization.

The main chemical reactions specifically for anodizing titanium are listed below (Equation (1) to (5) adapted from[4]).

At the Ti/Ti oxide interface:

$$Ti \Leftrightarrow Ti^{2+} + 2e^- \quad (1)$$

At the Ti oxide/electrolyte interface:

$$2H_2O \Leftrightarrow 2O^{2-} + 4H^+ \quad (2)$$

$$2H_2O \Leftrightarrow O_2 + 4H^+ + 4e^- \quad (3)$$

At both interfaces:

$$Ti^{2+} + 2O^{2-} \Leftrightarrow TiO_2 + 2e^- \quad (4)$$

Because titanium oxides have higher resistivity than the electrolyte and the metallic substrate, the applied voltage will mainly drop over the oxide film on the anode. As long as the electrical field is strong enough to drive the ion conduction through the oxide, the oxide film will keep growing. This explains why the final oxide thickness, d, is almost linearly dependent on the applied voltage, U:

$$d \approx aU \quad (5)$$

where a is usually a constant within the range 1.5-3 nm/V.[4]

2.2. Influences of Processing Parameters

The resulting oxide film properties (such as degree of nanometer roughness, morphology, chemistry, etc.) after anodization varies over a wide range according to different process parameters such as applied potential (voltage), current density, electrolyte composition, pH, and temperature. Different acids (phosphoric acid-H_3PO_4, sulfuric acid-H_2SO_4, acetic acid-CH_3COOH, and others), neutral salts, and alkaline solutions are widely-used electrolytes for the anodization of titanium. Their detailed electrochemical oxide growth behavior on titanium was studied by Sul et al.[16] Generally, it was found that among all the electrolytes (including H_3PO_4, H_2SO_4, CH_3COOH, and NaOH, $Ca(OH)_2$) the anodic oxide thickness in H_2SO_4 was the highest. Importantly, the oxide formation ability in acidic electrolytes exceeded that in hydroxide solutions. Usually, H_3PO_4 and H_2SO_4 were used to produce thick (tens of microns) and micro-porous oxide layers at high voltages. In contrast, fluoride solutions were found to have the ability of producing biologically-inspired nano-tubular structures in the past few years.[30-38] Due to the importance of nanostructures for biological applications as discussed above, this will be discussed in section 2.2.2.

The anodization process can be done either at constant voltage (poteniostatic) or constant current (galvanostatic). If the applied voltage exceeds the dielectric breakdown limit of the oxide, the oxide will no longer be resistive to prevent further current flow and oxide growth, which will lead to more gas revolution and sparking. This technique is, thus, known as Anodic Spark Deposition (ASD) or Micro-Arc Oxidation (MAO). For example, it has been reported that the breakdown potentials for H_3PO_4 and H_2SO_4 were around 80 and 100 V, respectively.[17] Below the breakdown limit, the anodic oxide film was relatively thin and usually non-porous using non-fluorine electrolytes.

A constant temperature during the anodization process is usually required to maintain a homogeneous field-enhanced dissolution over the entire area. Since increased temperature will accelerate the chemical dissolution rate, the working temperature is often kept relatively low to prevent the oxide from totally dissolving.[17]

2.3. Creation of Micron-Rough Surface

The anodization technique was discovered in the early 1930's and was widely studied in the 1960's to enhance titanium implant osseointegration.[18] These studies usually adopted a high voltage anodization (i.e., ASD) of titanium in electrolyte solutions whose ions would be embedded into the oxide coating, resulting in a micro-porous structure.[18-22, 24-27] Table 1 shows the anodizing parameters of some ASD studies.

The mechanism of the ASD is usually described by the avalanche theory. During anodization, the newly-formed oxide layer on the anode is a dielectric barrier to the current flow and it keeps growing until reaching the dielectric breakdown limit. Generally, the anodized layer is not

Table 1. Experimental parameters of some ASD studies.

Electrolyte Composition	Molarity	Voltage (Current)	Time (s)	Temp (°C)	Ref
Sulfuric acid	1	125	-	-	19
	0.5, 1, 3	90, 155, 180	-	-	20
Acetic acid	1	80	-	RT	21
	0.1	40-80	8-67	17	16
Phosphoric acid	2	175	-	25	19
	0.2	200, 300, 350 (70 A/cm^2)	-	20	22
	1	40-80	10-47	17	16
Sodium tripolyphosphate	0.15	(210 A/cm^2)	-	-	18
Sodium hydroxide	5	10-20	-	25	23
	0.1	40-80	22-110	17	16
Calcium hydroxide	0.1	40-80	13-53	17	16
Calcium glycerophosphate and calcium acetate	0.02/0.1	(70 A/cm^2)	1530	4.1-4.5	18
	0.03/0.15	200, 260, 300 (70 A/cm^2)		20	22
	0.15/0.02	190-600	180	-	24
	0.02/0.15	(70 A/cm^2)	1800	-	25
	0.02/0.15	350	1200	20	26
β glycerophosphate and sodium acetate	0.06/0.3	250-350 (50 A/cm^2)	-	-	27

RT = room temperature

uniform due to the existence of flaws, defects, local stress, and non-uniform oxide thickness. When the applied voltage increases, the potential drop at the weak points exceeds the dielectric limit so that sparking happens. The local temperature at these points can be up to several thousand Kelvin and lead to a local melting process. Thermal stressing of these anodized titanium leads to the multiplication of weak points, i.e., a cascading process, and consequently breakdown of the dielectric. Figure 2 shows a schematic diagram of porous titanium oxide formation proposed by Choi et al.[17]

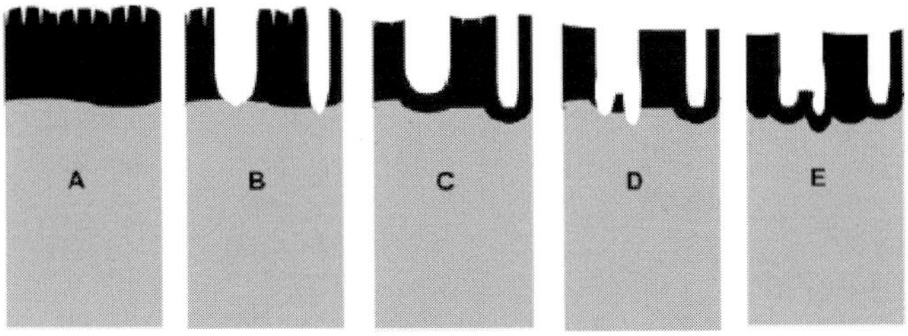

Figure 2. Schematic diagram of porous titanium oxide formation above the breakdown potential: (A) oxide growth to maximal thickness, (B) burst of oxide by the formation of crystallites (pore formation), (C) immediate repassivation of pore tips, (D) burst of repassivated oxide, and (E) dissolution of the formed oxide and second repassivation. (Adapted from[17])

Basically, the anodic film growth is determined by a balance between the oxide film formation rate and the oxide dissolution rate given by the nature of the electrolyte. Meanwhile, the nature of the electrolyte is closely connected with other processing parameters such as electrolyte concentration, applied voltage, current density, pH, etc. The explanations in detail could be found elsewhere.[16]

2.4. Creation of Nano-roughness

While the generation of micro-structures through titanium anodization is well-established, current research efforts focus on creating biologically-inspired nanometer surface structures. Studies has shown that nanoporous structures can be created by titanium anodization in chromic acid at 10 – 40 V.[28] Another unique surface morphologie obtained through titanium anodization is self-ordered nano-tubular structures.[30-38] For these studies, fluorine electrolyte solutions are used and the applied voltage must be much lower than the dielectric breakdown. Some of the specific anodizing parameters to create titanium nanometer structures are listed in Table 2.

Table 2. Survey of different fluorine solutions to produce titania nano-tubular structures with different size and thickness.

Electrolyte Composition (pH)	Voltage (V)	Time (h)	Temp. (°C)	Thickness (nm)	Pore diameter (nm)	Ref
CH_3COOH and 0.5 M HF	10	4	-	60	500 (inter)	17
0.5 or 1.5% HF	10-40	<1	18	250	25-65	30
0.5% HF	10-23	<1	-	300	22-76	31
KF and NaF (4.5)	25	20	-	4400	115	34
DMSO and CH_3COOH and 4% HF	20	70	RT	2300	60	35
1 M H_2SO_4 and 0.15% HF	30	24	-	540	140	32
CH_3COOH and 0.5% NH_4F	20	1	-	200	30	33
1 M $(NH_4)_2SO4$ and 0.5% NH_4F	20	-	-	2500	100	36
1 M $(NH_4)H_2PO_4$ and 1M H_3PO_4 and 0.5% HF	20	40	-	4070	50	37
0.138 M HF or NaF + 0.5 M H_3PO_4	20	-	24	500	100-120 (outer)	38

RT = room temperature

The need of fluoride ions to form nano-porous titania structures on a titanium surface under relatively low voltages was first reported by Zwilling et al.[29] However, the nano-tubular structures were not reported here. In 1999, Grimes and co-workers successfully fabricated self-ordered nano-tube arrays after anodizing titanium between 10 and 40 V in dilute (0.5-1.5 wt%) aqueous HF solutions.[30] It was found that the diameters of nano-tubes were determined by applied voltage while the final length of tubes were independent of the anodization time. The tube diameter was approximately 60 nm and tube length was 200 nm at 20 V in 0.5% HF solution for 20 min (Fig. 3). Later, they developed a method to produce tapered, conical-shape titania nano-tubes in 0.5% HF by linearly changing the voltage from 10 to 23 V (Fig. 4).[31] Schmuki and

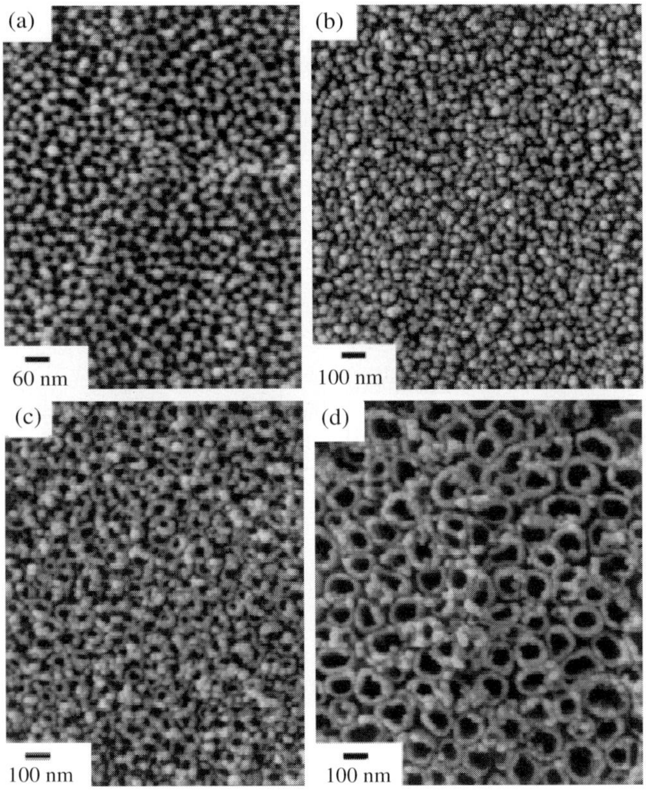

Figure 3. FE-SEM top-view images of porous titanium oxide films anodized in 0.5 wt% HF solution for 20 min under different voltages: (a) 3 V, (b) 5 V, (c) 10 V, and (d) 20 V. (Adapted from[30]).

co-workers also observed self-ordered nano-tubular titanium oxide films in HF/H_2SO_4 or CH_3COOH/NH_4F electrolyte solutions.[32] Moreover, the nano-tubular (nano-pore) structure was also achieved in organic electrolytes. Choi et al. used nano-indented titanium for anodization in ethanolic HF and produced a pore lattice with a 500 nm inter-pore distance (Fig. 5).[17] Schmuki's group reported nano-tubular structures using non-aqueous mixtures of ethanol and ammonium fluoride without an imprinting treatment.[33] However, in these studies, the depth of titania

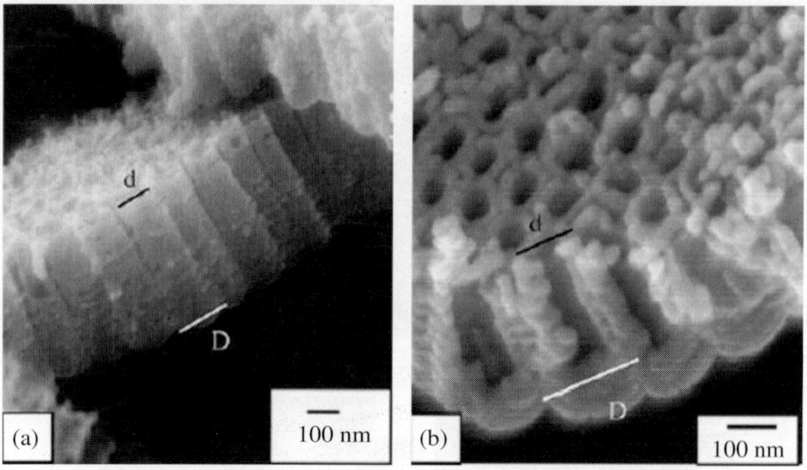

Figure 4. FE-SEM cross-sectional views of the titania nano-tubes obtained by using a time-varying anodization voltages; *d* denotes diameter of apex and *D* diameter of cone base. (a) Tapered nano-tubes obtained using a ramp rate of 0.43 V/min to raise the voltage from 10–23 V within 30 min and then holding the voltage at 23 V for 10 min. (b) Tapered nano-tubes obtained by initially anodizing the sample at 10 V for 20 min and then increasing the voltage linearly at a rate of 1.0 V/min to 23 V, and finally keeping the voltage at 23 V for 2 min (Adapted from[31]).

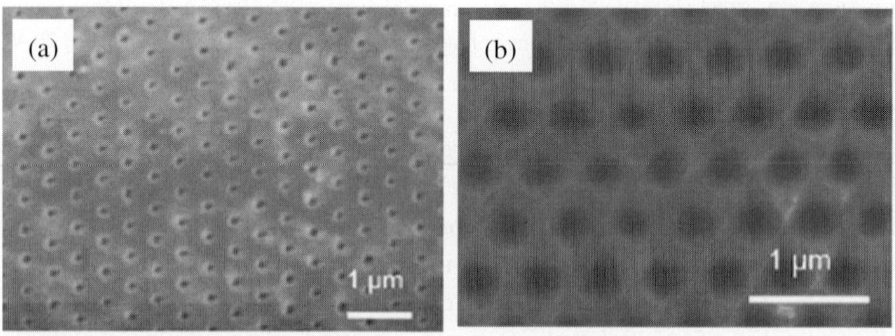

Figure 5. SEM of (a) nano-indented surface of titanium substrate and (b) anodized titanium at 10 V in ethanolic 0.5 M HF for 240 min. (Adapted from[17])

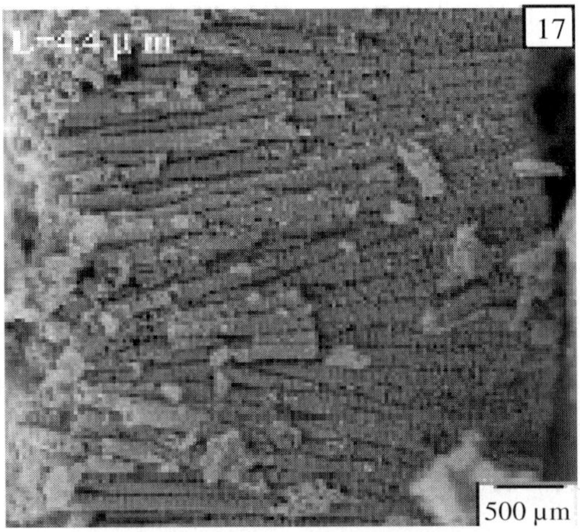

Figure 6. Lateral view of the nano-tubes formed in a KF and NaF solution at pH 4.5 under 25 V for 20 h. (Adapted from[34])

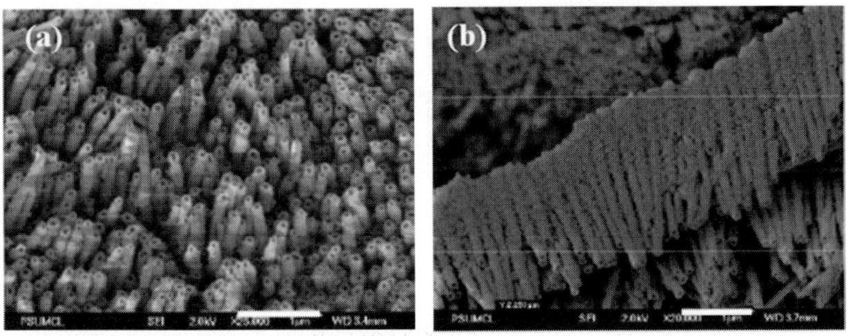

Figure 7. FE-SEM images of titanium foil sample anodized in DMSO and ethanol mixture solution (1:1) containing 4% HF at 20 V for 70 h. (a) is top-view and (b) is cross-section. Scale bars = 1 μm. (Adapted and redrawn from [35])

nano-tubes was limited to a few hundred of nanometers. Recently, high-aspect-ratio titania nano-tubes up to several micrometers were reported by both Grime's and Schmuki's groups.[34-37] Grime's group reported the formation of 4.4 μm long titania tube arrays by anodizing titanium in NaF or KF of pH 4.5 (Fig. 6).[34] They also reported formation of 2.3 μm thick nano-tubular structures using DMSO/ethanol/HF electrolyte (Fig. 7).[35] Meanwhile, Schmuki's group succeeded in using neutral fluoride solutions to produce nano-tubular structures up to 2.5 μm.[36] They achieved this by controlling the electrochemical parameters to enhance acidification at the bottom of tubes.

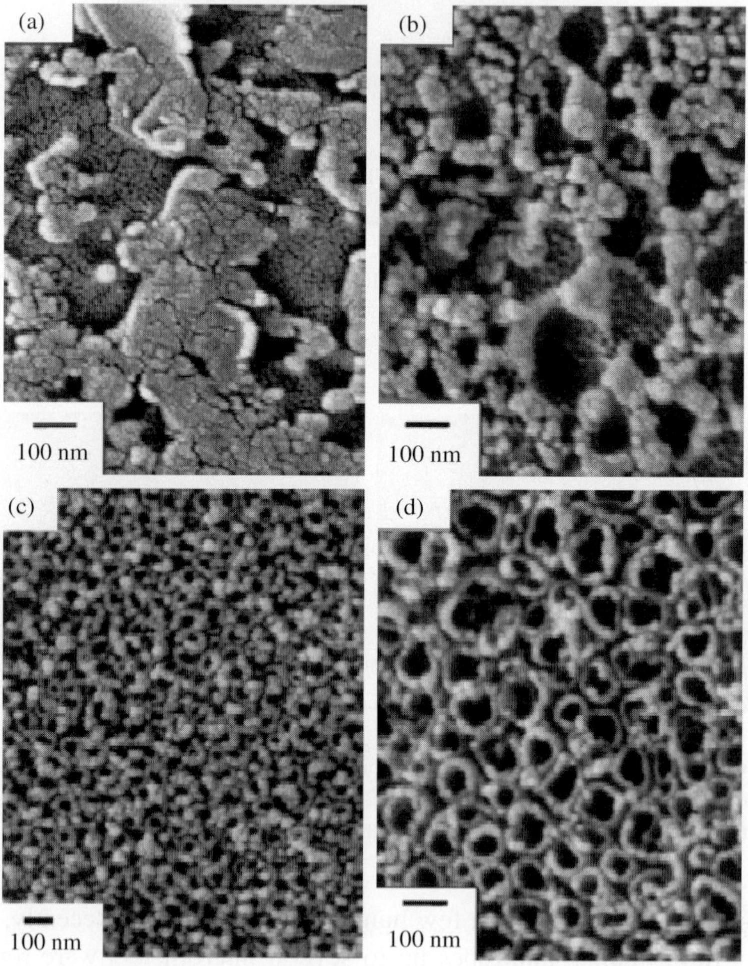

Figure 8. Evolution of nano-tube structures. Porous titanium oxide films anodized in 1.5% HF at 20 V for (a) 10s, (b) 30s, (c) 120s, and (d) 8 min. (Adapted from[30])

Chemical dissolution, field-assisted dissolution and oxidation are the three main reactions in fluorine electrolyte anodization. Among these, field-enhanced dissolution has been considered as the predominant mechanism of titania tubular structure formation by many researchers.[30-37] The evolution of nano-tube structures is shown in Fig. 8. Grime and co-workers proposed a mechanism based on a point defect model.[31] They proposed that the initial pore formation was due to localized dissolution at weak points and the unanodized metallic portions would exist between the pores. Later, voids were formed in these inter-pore regions by field-enhanced oxidation/dissolution (Fig. 9). The growth of voids in equilibrium with the pores would form the final nano-tubular structures. However, it didn't explain how voids can be created and lead pores to be well-separated, individual tubes. Recently, Raja et al. suggested that the instability of the oxide layer and the self-ordered structures could be explained by the perturbation theory; separation of individual nano-tubes of titanium oxide layer from the inter-connected nano-pores could be attributed to the repulsion forces of the cation vacancies (Fig. 10).[38]

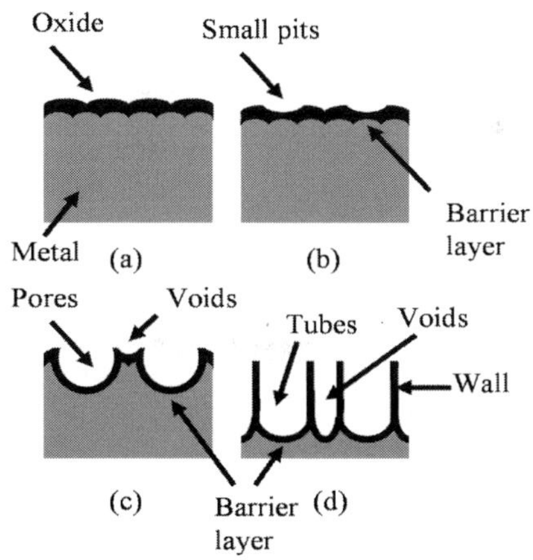

Figure 9. Schematic diagram of the evolution of nano-tube-like structures on the titanium surface during anodization in aqueous HF under constant voltage: (a) oxide formation; (b) pit formation in some concave sites; (c) pore formation and growth under field-enhanced dissolution leading to voids formation; and (d) fully developed tubes. (Based on the model from[31] and modified according to experimental observations).

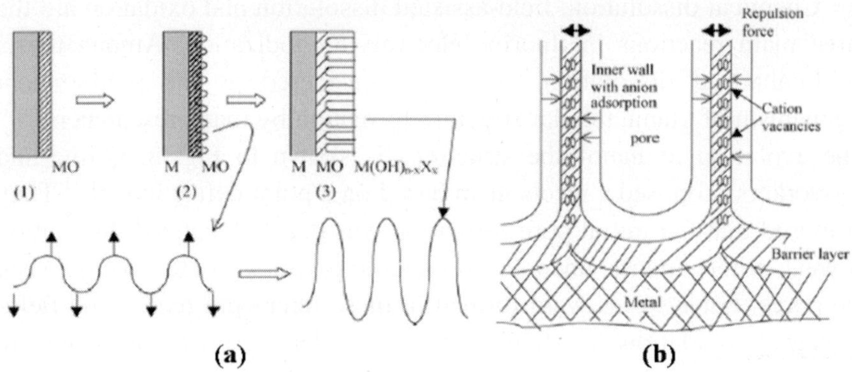

Figure 10. Schematic diagram of (a) pore formation (fluoride addition) during anodization of Ti. The barrier film is intact during porous anodic film formation and substrate metal is not attacked locally. Perturbation of the surface shown in (2) can lead to adsorption of fluorides at the valleys and develop into nano-tubular structure. Higher strain energy density at the valleys drives the mass flow to the lower energy crests; (b) pore separation mechanism. Cation vacancies generated by dissolution of Ti cations are transported radially from the two sides of common wall of the neighbor pores. Charges of similar polarity repel and when electrical neutrality is not maintained this repulsion causes separation of pores into individual nano-tubes. (Adapted and redrawn from[38])

2.5. Control of Chemical Composition

The ions contained in the electrolyte are usually present in the thick, porous ASD film and the concentration of these elements decreases from the outer layer towards the substrate.[22] For example, phosphorous was found to be embedded in titanium oxide layer after anodization with a H_3PO_4 electrolyte.[39] For electrolytes containing Ca and P, such as calcium glycerophosphate (Ca-GP) and calcium acetate (CA), both Ca and P were contained in the oxide layer with a Ca/P ratio close to HA (1.67).[40] After an additional hydrothermal treatment (e.g., high pressure streaming), HA crystals were randomly precipitated on the anodic oxide film. These HA crystals were usually columnar or need-like (Fig. 11). This could be another way to create HA coatings as opposed to plasma spraying. The advantages of such HA coatings compared to plasma sprayed HA will be discussed in following sections.

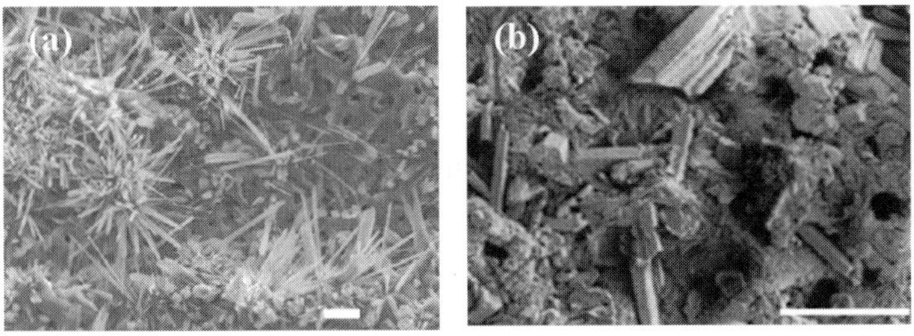

Figure 11. Needle-like or columnar hydroxyapatite crystals deposited on anodized titanium after a hydrothermal treatment. (a) ASD followed by Ishizawa's procedure[44] (Adapted and redrawn from[18]) and (b) ASD followed by Suh's procedure[25] (Adapted and redrawn from[25]). Scale bars = 10 μm.

Another approach reported to introduce apatite layers onto the anodized titanium is simply by soaking crystalline titania in simulated body fluid (SBF) because anodized titanium with anatase and rutile titania surfaces were shown to induce apatite formation in vitro. Yang et al. soaked titanium metal in SBF for 6 days after H_2SO_4 anodization and observed uniform apatite formation (Fig. 12).[20] One advantage of this method is that the composition and surface morphology of the resulting apatite layer is very close to those in natural bone, but the adhesive strength of such coatings are not clear yet.

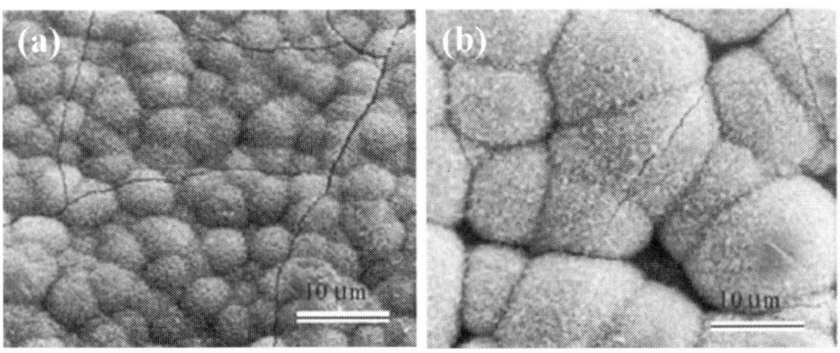

Figure 12. SEM images of titanium metal soaked in SBF for 6 days after they were anodized in 1 M H_2SO_4 at (a) 155 V and (b) 180 V. (Adapted and redrawn from[20])

Similarly, a two-step procedure was used to produce nano-scale HA for anodized titanium with nano-tubular structures.[41] Specifically, the anodized titanium was treated with NaOH to form nano-fibers of bioactive sodium titanate structures on the top edge of the nano-tube wall, which was then immersed in a SBF to induce the formation of nano-scale HA (Fig. 13). This technique could be useful as well-adherent bioactive nano-HA layers on titanium-based implants are created which simulate the size and shape of natural HA in bone. The advantage of introducing nano-HA onto titanium anodized structures was supported by previous work revealing greater osteoblast functions on nano-HA compared to conventional, or micron grain size, HA.[14]

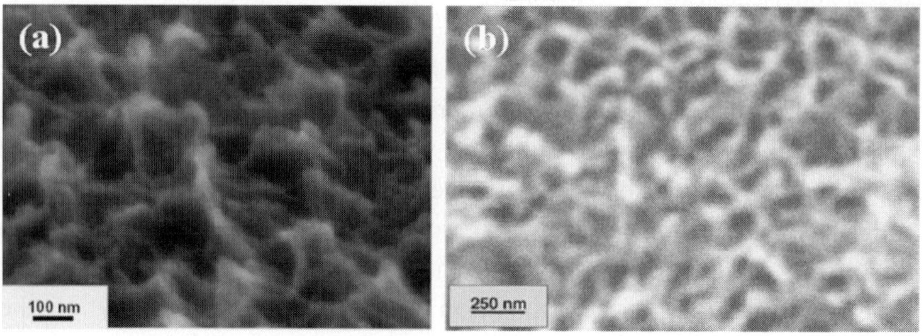

Figure 13. SEM images of (a) nano-inspired sodium titanate nano-fibers and (b) nanoscale HA phase. (Adapted and redrawn from[41])

3. Structure and Properties of Anodized Oxide Film

3.1. Structure

The structures and properties of ASD films were widely investigated by Kurze et al.[39] The typical morphology of the titania layer resulting from ASD is a rough, porous texture with cracks on it (Fig. 14 and 15). The dimensions of the pores varied from a few hundred nanometers to a few micrometers depending on the processing parameters and are not uniform within the same anodized surface. Moreover, these pores were interconnected and had a layered structure, i.e., they overlapped with each other. The shapes of the pores were mostly round or irregular. The diameter of the pores and the film roughness were reported to increase with greater current densities (Fig. 14),[18, 42] applied potential (Fig. 15),[20] and electrolyte concentrations.[20] The thickness of oxide film increases with time up to tens of micrometers.

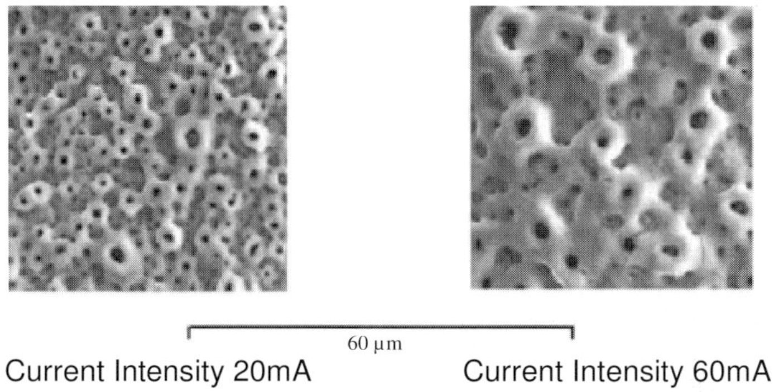

Figure 14. SEM micrographs of an ASD formed film on c.p. grade 2 titanium from an electrolyte containing 0.015 M calcium glycerophosphate and 0.1 M calcium acetate. Increased current density from 20 to 60 mA/cm^2 led to a larger pore size in the ASD porous structure (Adapted from[18]).

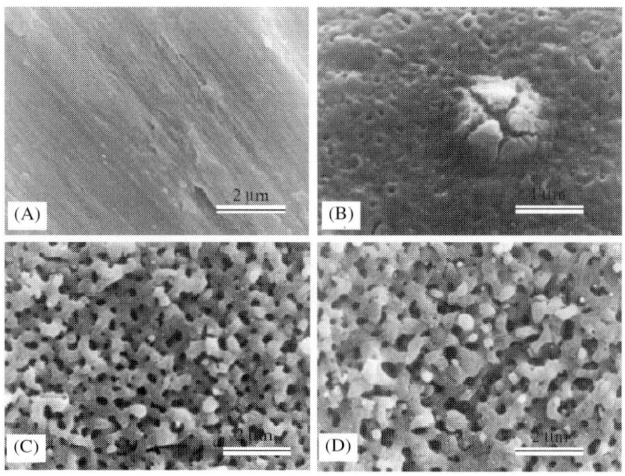

Figure 15. SEM micrographs of ASD formed film on c.p. titanium from an electrolyte containing 1 M H_2SO_4 at voltages of: (a) 0 V, (b) 90V, (c) 155 V, and (d) 180 V for 1 min. Different voltages from 90 to 155 V led to a larger pore size in the ASD porous structure (Adapted from[20]).

In contrast, the biological-inspired nano-tubular structures were highly ordered. The pore size is determined by the voltage and can be varied from a few tens of nanometers to around 100 nanometers. The thickness of the tubular-structured oxide was formed to be a few hundred nanometers but has been elongated to a few microns by controlling pH and electrolytes. Generally, the dimensions of nano-tubular structures within one sample are uniform but might be variable due to differences (e.g., surface defects) on a substrate.

3.2. Corrosion Resistance and Adhesive Strength

After anodization, thickness of the protective oxide layer increases and it could lead to less ion release in the human body. The oxide barrier layer (the relatively thin, non-porous oxide layer under the porous oxide structures) is considered to contribute to the improvement of corrosion resistance. However, it was suggested that the implants' mechanical properties could be impaired with increased spark coating thickness.[18]

The interface between the anodic oxide layer and the titanium substrate usually does not show any discontinuity.[18] Besides, the HA crystals on the hydrothermally treated titanium are gradually grown consuming Ca and P in the anodic film. As a result, the interface between the substrate, the anodic film, and the HA film are considerably strong.
The adhesive strength between the anodic oxide films and the titanium substrates was reported to be 25 MPa,[43] and the adhesive strength between the oxide/HA coating and the substrate after a hydrothermal treatment was reported to be up to 40 MPa by Ishizawa et al. when using less concentrated electrolytes.[40, 44] These values are equivalent or higher than those of plasma sprayed HA onto titanium surfaces, which were reported between 15 to 30 MPa depending on different processing parameters.[45,46] Moreover, the HA produced from hydrothermal treatment after anodization (AH-HA) seemed to be more stable than plasma sprayed HA (PS-HA). It was reported that the shear strength of PS-HA in SBF decreased from 28.1 MPa to 20.4 MPa after 4 weeks[47]; meanwhile, Ishizawa et al. found that AH-HA retained high durability after 300 days in SBF.[40] So from a mechanical point-of-view,

hydrothermally treated anodic titanium would be a better choice than HA plasma sprayed titanium.

3.3. Biological Properties of Anodized Titanium

3.3.1. In vitro Studies

Clearly, coating strength, mechanical and other properties are not the only concern for orthopedic implants. Cytocompatibility leading to promoted bone growth needs to be assessed. Most studies have been reported in vitro bone cell responses to anodized and anodized / hydrothermally treated titanium surface. Fini et al. reported that the adhesion, spreading, proliferation, and differentiation of osteoblast-like cells (HOS-TE85, human osteosarcoma line) were similar on unanodized titanium, titanium anodized enriched with Ca/P, and titanium anodized and hydrothermally treated.[27] An unexpected increase of unattached cells in the latter two substrates was observed. However, the percentage of unattached cells was in the range of 10-20% which is considered a normal range for cytocompatible materials. On contrast, Rodriguez et al. reported increased osteocalcin production on the anodized and hydrothermally treated titanium surfaces but the highest alkaline phosphate (ALP) activity on control titanium throughout an 8 day study using an osteoblast precursor cell line (ATCC, CRL-1468).[48] Both osteocalcin and ALP are markers of osteoblast differentiation to deposit calcium. They explained that a decrease in ALP activity was in part attributed to the maturation of osteoblast precursor cells and in part attributed to the increased production of mineralized matrix. Also using Ca-GP and CA as an electrolyte, Li et al. reported decreased osteoblastic MG63 cell proliferation when anodization voltage increased above 190 V; however, increased ALP activity of human osteosarcoma cell line was reported with voltages above 300 V.[24]

Zhu et al. studied the effects of topography and composition of anodized titanium surfaces on osteoblast (SaOS-2 derived from human osteosarcoma) responses.[22] Their cell experiments showed an absence of cytotoxicity and an increase of cell attachment and proliferation after anodization in an electrolyte composed of Ca-GP and CA. The cells on the surfaces with micro-pores showed an irregular and polygonal growth and more lamellipodia while cells on the titanium control showed many thick stress fibers and intense focal contacts. However, they didn't find any significant difference for ALP activity. Suh et al. studied the effects of hydrothermally treated anodic films similar to the Zhu formulations and they observed no statistical differences in cell viability using the MTT assay when osteoblasts (ROS 17/2.8, a rat osteosarcoma cell line) were cultured for 4 days on untreated, anodized, and anodized / hydrothermally treated surfaces.[25] In contrast, they found that hydrothermal treatment had an effect on early osteoblast attachment, resulting in a more well-spread shape compared to the cellular rounded shape observed on anodized and control titanium after 6 h (Fig. 16).

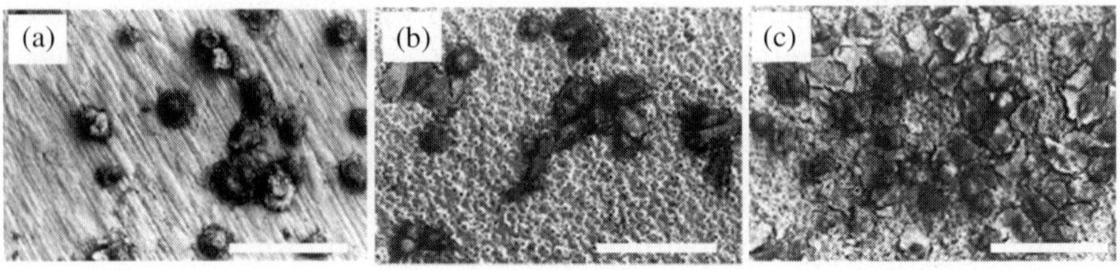

Figure 16. SEM of cells after 6 h culturing on (a) control surface, (b) anodized surface and (c) anodized surface followed by hydrothermal treatment for 4 h. Scale bars = 120 μm. (Adapted from[25])

The different observations in the above in vitro studies could be attributed to the use of different anodization parameters and different cell lines. The optimal anodization conditions are still under investigation.

Since the nano-tubular structure is relatively new, few cytocompatibility studies have been completed to examine its potential for use as a novel titanium bone implant surface. However, because of the size and order of the titania tubular structure (which somewhat mimics the natural environment of bone) it is very interesting to determine whether there is any morphological or size advantage of using nano-tubular structures compared to a conventional anodized titanium porous structure for enhancing bone cell functions.

Currently, our research has focused on osteoblast functions on such anodized titanium with nano-tubular titania structures. These structures are similar to those formed by Gong et al.[30] (0.5% HF, 20 V, 20 min). After anodization, the tubular structures had increased surface roughness (Fig. 17). The inner diameters of the nano-tubes were about 70 nm and the depth of them was about 200 nm. To study the effects of nanoroughness and morphology, intermediate samples that possessed a nano-particulate structure and a medium roughness in between the unanodized control and the nano-tubular structure were created (0.5% HF, 10 V, 20 min) (Fig. 17).

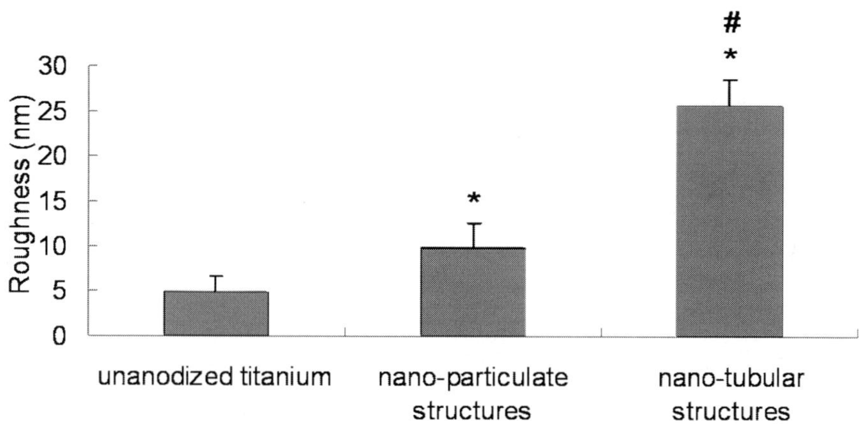

Figure 17. Surface roughness of (a) unanodized titanium, (b) anodized titanium with nano-particulate structures, and (c) anodized titanium with nano-tubular structures. Data = mean ± SEM; n = 3; *$p < 0.01$ (compared to unanodized titanium) and #$p < 0.01$ (compared to nano-particulate structure).

The experiments showed increased osteoblast adhesion after 4 hour of culture with greater anodized titanium roughness (Fig. 18). The difference in osteoblast morphology was obvious between nano-tubular structures and unanodized titanium. Most cells were well-spread on anodized titanium with nano-tubular structures while they mostly looked round on the control (Fig. 19). After 4 weeks of culture, the anodized titanium with nano-tubular structures promoted the highest calcium deposition by osteoblasts among all the samples. These results indicated that the special nano-tubular structures anodized onto the titanium surface may have provided an optimal surface roughness for promoting bone cell function.

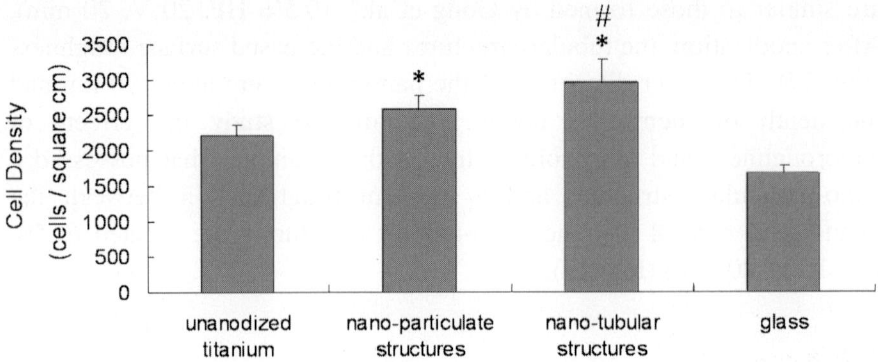

Figure 18. Osteoblast adhesion on unanodized titanium, anodized titanium with nano-particulate structures (10 V, 0.5% HF, 20 min), anodized titanium with nano-tubular structures (20 V, 0.5% HF, 20 min), and glass (reference). Values are mean ± SEM; n = 3; *p < 0.1 (compared to unanodized titanium) and #p < 0.1 (compared to anodized titanium with nano-particulate structures).

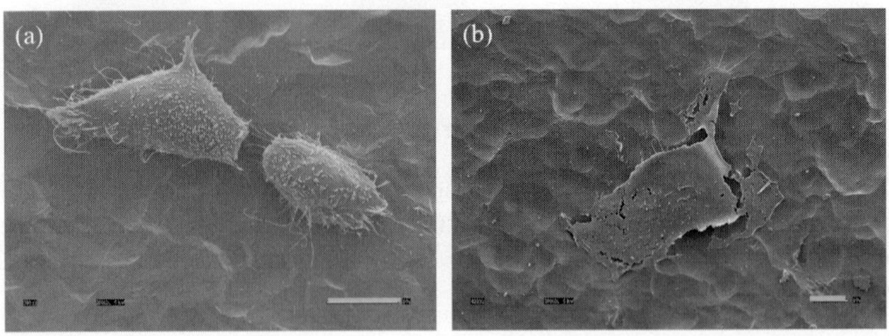

Figure 19. Typical osteoblast morphology on (a) unanodized titanium and (b) anodized titanium surface with nano-tubular structures after 4 h culture. Scale bars = 10 μm.

3.3.2. Mechanisms of Increased Osteoblast Function

Moreover, protein (fibronectin and vitronectin) adsorption on nano-tubular samples has been examined to explore the mechanism of enhanced osteoblast adhesion. Fibronectin and vitronectin are two major proteins that involved in osteoblast adhesion.[49-51] Results showed significantly increased both fibronectin (15%) and vitronectin (18%) adsorption on nano-tubular structures compared to unanodized titanium samples (Fig. 20). Because the cells adhered to the titanium surface via pre-adsorbed proteins, increased fibronectin and vitronectin adsorption on anodized titanium substrates with nano-tubular structures may explain the observed enhanced osteoblast functions.

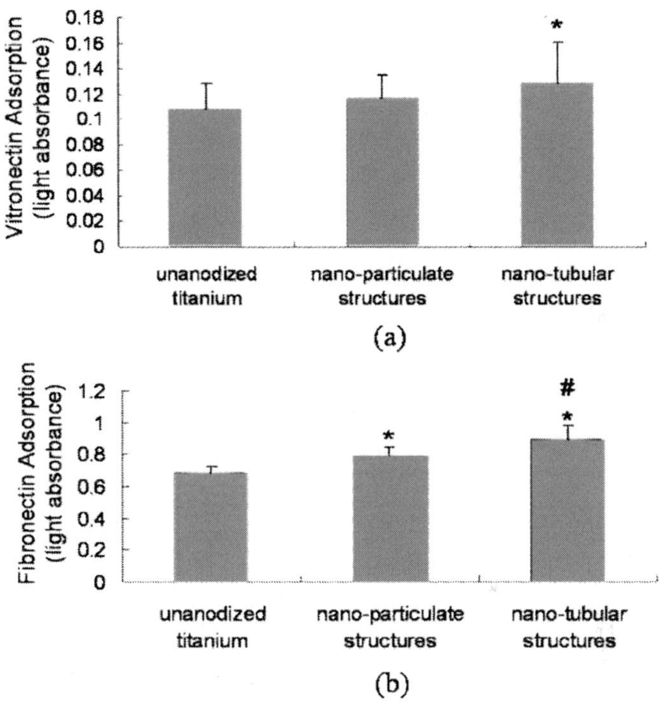

Figure 20. (a) Fibronectin and (b) vitronectin adsorption on unanodized titanium, anodized titanium possessing nano-particulate structures (0.5% HF, 10 V and 20 min), and anodized titanium possessing nano-tubular structures (0.5% HF, 20 V and 20 min). Values are mean ± SEM; n = 3; *p < 0.1 (compared to unanodized titanium) and #p < 0.1 (compared to nano-particulate structures).

3.3.3. In vivo Studies

While in vitro assays may generate a quick assessment of cytocompatibility, in vivo studies are necessary to fully evaluate new bone growth. A survey of in vivo investigations of bone tissue reactions to anodized titanium implants is listed in Table 3. As with in vitro analysis, the varied oxide properties not only include thickness, but also morphology, chemical composition, crystallinity, and surface roughness.

Some in vivo studies were mainly interested in the effects of thick, porous oxide coating on new bone growth. Less than 200 nm thick oxide film anodized in acetic acid showed no significant difference compared to unanodized samples after implanted into a rabbit 6 weeks.[21] In contrast, a H_3PO_4/H_2SO_4 electrolyte was usually used to form thick anodic films up to tens of microns. Enhanced bone bonding was found for micron-thick porous anodic oxide films formed in a H_3PO_4/H_2SO_4 electrolyte solution in a rabbit model.[52-54]

More importantly, changes of surface chemistry could play a more important role in inducing new bone growth. Several in vivo studies focused on Ca-P enriched anodized titanium with and without hydrothermal treatment.[24,27,55-58] Ishizawa et al. produced 1-2 μm HA films on anodic oxide layer and compared bone growth on them with unanodized titanium.[55] They found strong bone bonding via push-out tests with anodized titanium after 8 weeks of implantation into rabbits. Following their in vitro work, Fini et al. found the lowest affinity index on anodized titanium while the highest was found on the anodized and hydrothermally treated titanium.[27] The low bone contact on anodized titanium was probably due to the in vivo reduction and degradation of the amorphous titania layer while HA crystals aided bone opposition. Giavaresi et al. also supported the positive role of HA produced from hydrothermal treatment in accelerating bone ingrowth and bone mineralization.[56-57] Son et al. reported no significant difference for the percent bone contact for all samples but did find significantly increased removal torque strength for anodized implants after 6 weeks of implantation into a rabbit.[58]

The dissolution of AH-HA and PS-HA in vivo was studied by Ishizawa et al.[59] Basically, the AH-HA was much more durable than PS-HA because of their relatively high crystallinity and their relatively low thickness. Ishizawa et al. also found these two HA had different bone responses.[59] Specifically, new bone thinly spread over the whole AH-HA area while new bone formed from surrounding bones to the PS-HA area. This is probably due to their different degradation properties.

Table 3. Survey of in vivo investigations of bone tissue reactions to anodized titanium implants.

Implant	Treatment	Chemical composition	Oxide thickness (μm)	Oxide / HA morphology (pore size, μm)	Oxide / HA crystallinity	Roughness (μm)	Test	Animal and time (week)	Reference
Cylinder	AO and HT	TiO_2, HA	< 10	Porous (1-3)	A+R	ND	Push-out	Rabbits 8	55
Screw	E/M and AO	Mainly TiO_2	0.18-0.2	Pores and pits	N	32.3/40.8 nm (rms)	contact ratio	Rabbits 1, 3, 6	21
Screw	AO	Ti, O, C, P/S	1/10	Porous (1-10)	A+R	1.2 (Sa)	RTQ, RFA	Rabbits 3, 6	52
Rod	Ca-P AO w/ or w/o HT	Ti, O, Ca/P, HA	5	porous (1-3) / columnar	N / C	1.97 (Ra)	AI	Rats 4, 8	27
Screw	Ca-P AO and HT	Ti, O, Ca/P, HA	ND	porous	ND	1.97 (Ra)	AI, push-out strength	Sheep 4, 8, 12	56, 57
Screw	Ca-P AO w/ or w/o HT	Ti, O, Ca/P, HA	ND	Porous / needle-like	A+R / C	ND	percent bone contact, RTQ	Rabbits 6,12	58
Screw	AO	Primary TiO_2	0.2-1	Porous (1.27-2.10)	N, A, A+R	0.96-1.04 (Sa)	RTQ, RFA	Rabbits 6	53, 54
Screw	AO	Ti, O, S, P, Ca	1.1-1.3	Porous (<1.5)	A or N	0.82-1.04 (Sa)	RTQ, BMC	Rabbits 6	60

Abbreviations: AO-anodization, HT-hydrothermal treatment, E-electropolished, M-machined. C-crystalline, N-noncrystalline, A-anatase, R-rutile, RTQ-removal torque values, RFA-resonance frequency analysis, AI-affinity index, BMC-bone to metal, ND-not determined.

One drawback of most of the above studies is that both chemical composition and surface morphology changed after titanium anodization so that it is hard to verify the role of one material property. However, Sul et al. indirectly verified a chemical bonding in vivo by maintaining surface morphology and roughness and changing chemical characteristics (specifically, S, P and Ca enriched implants via anodization).[60] The removal torque value (RTQ) showed significant differences between Ca-containing anodized titanium implants and unanodized titanium implants as well as S-containing anodized titanium implants and unanodized titanium implants (Fig. 21). The bone to metal contact was 186%, 232%, and 272% higher in S, P, and Ca implants, respectively, when compared to the control groups. These results confirmed that ions incorporated into the titanium oxide layer during anodization could have important roles in enhancing bone juxtaposition.

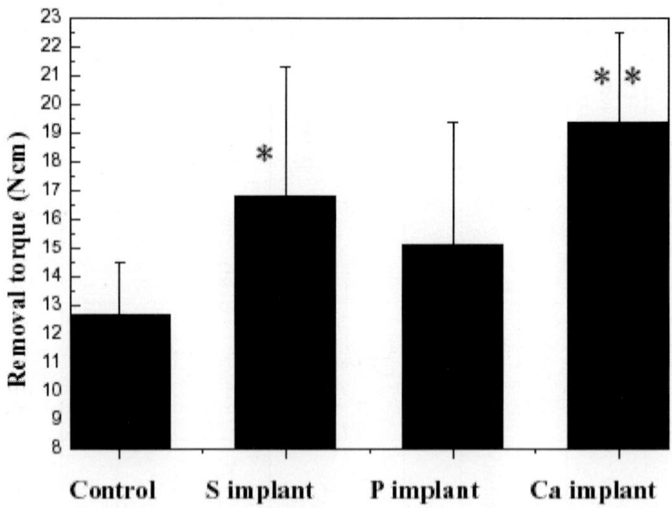

Figure 21. Mean removal torque values after 6 weeks of healing time. *p < 0.05, **p < 0.001. (Adapted from[60])

4. Future Directions

As a surface modification method, anodization can lead to desired chemistry and/or topography changes and could be used with other treatments (e.g., hydrothermal) together.

First, anodization provides a controlled way to create nano-roughness or even nano-features. Generally, there are two mechanisms that are responsible for osseointegration of bone: biomechanical interlocking and biological interactions. For biomechanical interlocking, it depends on the roughness, and surface irregularity. Current femoral stems made of titanium alloys are usually macro-textured to provide such surface features for bone to mechanically interlock. For biological interactions, it involves complex systems. Considering roughness in different scales, it is reported that increased micro/submicron-roughness could enhance bone cell function, such as ALP activity.[61,62] while some other studies have revealed the enhanced cell-implant interactions on nanoporous or nanophase materials.[14,15,63,64] Ideally, the future titanium implant should possess roughness in all three scales: macro, micro, and nano. One possible approach to accomplish this is by subjecting implants to techniques like polishing and mechanical grinding that promote micro-roughness, and then to induce nano-tubular structures by a quick anodization process.

Second, micro/nano HA films produced using anodized titanium shows some advantages over conventional ones. Although plasma spray is still widely used for HA coatings on titanium, anodization has a strong role to play to incorporate Ca and P into Ti coatings. For example, anodization has the ability to form uniform and thin HA or calcium phosphate layers on titanium implants of various shapes. Moreover, HA deposited onto the anodized titanium could be nano-scale in dimension. One problem that still needs to be more fully investigated is the bonding strength between apatite crystals and the anodic oxide.

Furthermore, anodization can be used to incorporate drug delivery into titanium-based implants to enhance new bone formation. Porous ASD surfaces could be used as matrices for drug storage and release[65]; similarly, the nano-tubular structures could serve as reservoirs of chemical mediators, such as bone morphogenetic protein-2 (BMP-2) and osteogenic protein-1 (OP-1, BMP-7).[66] In the future, studies should concentrate on embedding these growth factors into the unique porosity that can be well controlled on titanium for orthopedic applications.

In a word, anodization as a quick and efficient modification method of titanium based implants shows significant promise for enhancing their 10 to 15 year lifetime.

Acknowledgements

The authors would like to thank National Science Foundation Nanoscale Exploratory Research Grant for financial assistance.

Bibliography

1. Brunette DM, Tengvall P, Textor M, and Thomsen P. (2001) Mechanical, thermal, chemical and electrochemical surface treatment of titanium. In *Titanium in Medicine* Thomsen P (ed.), Springer, New York, NY, p. 171.
2. Shackelford JF. (1999) *Bioceramics* Netherlands, Gordon and Breach Science Publishers, New York, NY, p. 17.
3. Moran CG, Horton TC. (2000) Total knee replacement: the joint of the decade. A successful operation, for which there's a large unmet need. *BMJ* **320**: 820.
4. Brunette DM, Tengvall P, Textor M, and Thomsen P. (2001) Mechanical, thermal, chemical and electrochemical surface treatment of titanium. In *Titanium in Medicine* Thomsen P (ed.), Springer, New York, NY, p. 232.
5. Larsson C, Thomsen P, Aronsson BO, Rodahl M, Lausmaa J, Kasemo B and Ericson LE. (1996) Bone response to surface-modified titanium implants: studies on the early tissue response to machined and electropolished implants with different oxide thicknesses. *Biomaterials* **17**: 605.
6. Kim HM, Miyaji F, Kokubo T, Nakamura T. (1997) Effect of heat treatment on apatite-forming ability of Ti metal induced by alkali treatment. *J. Mater. Sci.: Mater. Med.* **8**: 341.
7. Kokubo T, Kim HM, Kawashita M, Nakamura T. (2004) Bioactive metal: preparation and properties. *J. Mater. Sci.: Mater. Med.* **15**: 899.
8. Sittig C, Textor M, Spencer ND, Wieland M, Vallotton PH. (1999) Surface characterization of implant materials c.p. Ti, Ti-6Al-7Nb and Ti-6Al-4V with different pretreatments. *J. Mater. Sci.: Mater. Med.* **10**: 35.

9. Bordji K, Jouzeau JY, Mainard D, Payan E, Netter P, Rie KT, Stucky T and Hage-Ali M. (1996) Cytocompatibility of Ti-6Al-4V and Ti-5Al-2.5Fe alloys according to three surface treatments, using human fibroblasts and osteoblasts. *Biomaterials* **17**: 929.
10. Furlong R, Osborn JF. (2001) Fixation of hip prostheses by hydroxyapatite ceramic coatings. *J. Bone Joint Surg.* **73B**: 741.
11. Kim SS, Park MS, Jeon O, Choi CY and Kim BS. (2007) Poly(lactide-co-glycolide)/hydroxyapatite composite scaffolds for bone tissue engineering. *Biomaterials*, In Press.
12. Baker KC, Anderson MA, Oehlke SA, Astashkina AI, Haikio DC, Drelich J and Donahue SW. (2007) Growth, characterization and biocompatibility of bone-like calcium phosphate layers biomimetically deposited on metallic substrata. *Growth, Materials Science and Engineering*: *C* **26**: 1351.
13. Sato M, Slamovich EB and Webster TJ. (2005) Enhanced osteoblast adhesion on hydrothermally treated hydroxyapatite/titania/poly(lactide-co-glycolide) sol-gel titanium coatings. *Biomaterials* **26**: 1349.
14. Bronzino JD. (1995) *Biomedical Engineering Handbook.* CRC Press, New York, NY, p. 274.
15. Webster TJ, Ejiofor JU. (2004) Increased osteoblast adhesion on nanophase metals: Ti, Ti6Al4V, CoCrMo. *Biomaterials* **25**: 4731.
16. Sul YT, Johansson CB, Jeong Y, Albrektsson T. (2001) The electrochemical oxide growth behavior on titanium via acid and alkaline electrolytes. *Medical Engineering & Physics* **23**: 329.
17. Choi J, Wehrspohn RB, Lee J, Gosele U. (2004) Anodization of nanoimprinted titanium: a comparison with formation of porous alumina. *Electrochimica Acta* **49**: 2645.
18. Chiesa R, Sandrini E, Santin M, Rondelli G, Cigada A. (2003) Osteointegration of titanium and its alloys by anodic spark deposition and other electrochemical techniques: A review. *J. Applied Biomaterials & Biomechanics* **1**: 91.
19. Zinger O, Chauvy PF, Landolt D. (2003) Scale – resolved electrochemical surface structuring of titanium for biological applications. *J. of the Electrochemical Society* **150**: 495.
20. Yang B, Uchida M, Kim HM, Zhang X and Kokubo T. (2004) Preparation of bioactive titanium metal via anodic oxidation treatment. *Biomaterials* **25**: 1003.
21. Larsson C, Thomsen P, Aronsson BO, Rodahl M, Lausmaa J, Kasemo B and Ericson LE. (1996) Bone response to surface-modified titanium implants: studies on the early tissue response to machined and electropolished implants with different oxide thicknesses. *Biomaterials* **17**: 605.
22. Zhu X, Chen J, Scheideler C, Reichl R and Geis-Gerstorfer J. (2004) Effects of topography and composition of titanium surface oxides on osteoblast responses. *Biomaterials* **25**: 4087.

23. Huang HH, Pan SJ, Lai YL, Lee TH, Chen CC and Lu FH. (2004) Osteoblast-like cell initial adhesion onto a network-structured titanium oxide layer. *Scripta Materialia* **51**: 1017.
24. Li LH, Kong YM, Kim HW, Kim YW, Kim HE, Heo SJ and Koak JY. (2004) Improved biological performance of Ti implants due to surface modification by micro-arc oxidation. *Biomaterials* **25**: 2867.
25. Suh JY, Jang BC, Zhu X, Ong JL, and Kim K. (2003) Effect of hydrothermally treated anodic oxide films on osteoblast attachment and proliferation. *Biomaterials* **24**: 347.
26. Son WW, Zhu X, Shin HI, Ong JL, Kim KH. (2003) In vivo histological response to anodized and anodized/hydrothermally treated titanium implants. *J. Biomed. Mater. Res. Part B Appl. Biomater.* **66B**: 520.
27. Fini M, Cigada A, Rondelli G, Chiesa R, Giardino R, Giavaresi G, Aldini NN, Torricelli P, Vicentini B. (1999) In vitro and in vivo behaviour of Ca- and P-enriched anodized titanium. *Biomaterials* **20**: 1587.
28. Baun WL. (1980) Formation of porous films on titanium alloys by anodization. *Surf. Technol.* **11**: 421.
29. Zwilling V, Darque-Ceretti E, Boutry-Forveille A, David D, Perrin MY, Aucouturier M. (1999) Structure and physicochemistry of anodic oxide films on titanium and T4Al6V alloy. *Surf. Interface Anal.* **27**: 629.
30. Gong D, Grimes CA, Varghese OK, Hu W, Singh RS, Chen Z, and Dickey EC. (2001) Titanium oxide nanotube arrays prepared by anodic oxidation. *J. Mater. Res.* **16**: 3331.
31. Mor GK, Varghese OK, Paulose M, Mukherjee N, and Grimes CA. (2003) Fabrication of tapered, conical-shaped titania nanotubes. *J. Mater. Res.* **18**: 2588.
32. Beranek R, Hildebrand H, and Schmuki P. (2003) Self-organized porous titanium oxide prepared in H_2SO_4/HF electrolytes. *Electrochemical and solid-state letters* **6**: B12.
33. Tsuchiya H, Macak JM, Taveira L, Balaur E, Ghicov A, Sirotna K, Schmuki P. (2005) Self-organized TiO_2 nanotubes prepared in ammonium fluoride containing acetic acid electrolyte. *Electrochemistry communications* **7**: 576.
34. Cai Q, Paulose M, Varghese OK, and Grimes CA. (2005) The effect of electrolyte composition on the fabrication of self-organized titanium oxide nanotube arrays by anodic oxidation. *J. Mater. Res.* **20**: 230.
35. Ruan C, Paulose M, Varghese OK, Mor GK, and Grimes CA. (2005) Fabrication of highly ordered TiO_2 nanotube arrays using an organic electrolyte. *J. Phys. Chen. B* **109**: 15754.
36. Macak JM, Tsuchiya H, Schmuki P. (2005) High-aspect-ratio TiO_2 nanotubes by anodization of titanium. *Chem. Int. Ed.* **44**: 2100.
37. Ghicov A, Tsuchiya H, Macak JM, Schmuki P. (2005) Titanium oxide nantubes prepared in phosphate electrolyte. *Electrochemistry communications* **7**: 505.

38. Raja KS, Misra M, Paramguru K. (2005) Formation of self-ordered nanotubular structure of anodic oxide layer on titanium. *Electrochimica Acta* **51**: 154.
39. Kurze P, Krysmann W, Schneider HG. (1986) Application fields of ANOF layer and composites. *Cryst. Res. Technol.* **21**: 1603.
40. Ishizawa H, Ogino M. (1995) Mechanical and histological investigation of hydrothermally treated and untreated anodic titanium oxide films containing Ca and P. *J. Biomed. Mater. Res.* **29**: 1071.
41. Oh SH, Finõnes RR, Daraio C, Chen LH, and Jin S. (2005) Growth of nano-scale hydroxyapatite using chemically treated titanium oxide nanotubes. *Biomaterials* **26**: 4938.
42. Delplancke JL, Winand R. (1973) Galvanostatic anodization of titanium – I. Structures and Composition of the anodic films. *Electrochim Acta* **33**: 1539.
43. Schreckenback JP, Marx G, Schlottig F, Textor M, Spencer ND. (1999) Characterization of anodic spark converted titanium surfaces for biomedical applications. *Journal of Surface Science, Materials in Medicine* **10**: 453.
44. Ishizawa H, Ogino M. (1995) Formation and characterization of anodic titanium oxide films containing Ca and P. *J. Biomed. Mater. Res.* **29**: 65.
45. Lu YP, Zhu RF, Li ST, Song YJ, Li MS, Lei TQ. (2003) Plasma sprayed graded titanium hydroxyapatite coatings. *Materials Science and Technology* **19**: 260.
46. Yang Y, Ong JL. (2003) Bond strength, compositional, and structural properties of hydroxyapatite coating on Ti, ZrO2-coated Ti, and TPS-coated Ti substrate. *J. Biomed. Mater. Res. A* **64**: 509.
47. Yang YC, Chang E, Lee SY. (2003) Mechanical properties and Young's modulus of plasma sprayed hydroxyapatite coating on Ti substrate in simulated body fluid. *J. Biomed. Mater. Res. A* **67**: 886.
48. Rodriguez R, Kim K, Ong JL. (2003) In vitro osteoblast response to anodized titanium and anodized titanium followed by hydrothermal treatment. *J. Biomed. Mater. Res. A* **65**: 352.
49. Anselme K. (2000) Review: Osteoblast adhesion on biomaterials. *Biomaterials* **21**: 667.
50. Hayman EG, Pierschbacher MD, Suzuki S, Ruoslahti E. (1985) Vitronectin- a major cell attachment-promoting protein in feral bovine serum. *Exp. Cell Res.* **160**: 245.
51. Thomas CH, McFarland CD, Jenkins ML, Rezania A, Steel JC, Healy KE. (1997) The role of vitronectin in the attachment and spatial distribution of bone-derived cells on materials with patterned surface chemistry. *J. Biomed. Mater. Res.* **37**: 81.
52. Henry P, Tan AE, Allan BP. (2000) Removal torque comparison of Tiunite and turned implants in the Greyhound dog mandible. *APPL Osseointegration Res.* **1**: 15.
53. Sul YT, Johansson CB, Jeong Y, Wennerberg A, Albrektsson T. (2002) Resonance frequency and removal torque analysis of implants with turned and anodized surface oxide Clin. *Oral Implants Res.* **13**: 252.

54. Sul YT, Johansson CB, Roser K, Albrektsson T. (2002) Qualitative and quantitative observations of bone tissue reactions to anodized implants. *Biomaterials* **23**: 1809.
55. Ishizawa H, Fugino M, Ogino M. (1995) Mechanical and histological investigation of hydrothermally treated and untreated anodic titanium oxide films containing Ca and P. *J. Biomed. Mater. Res.* **29**: 1459.
56. Giavaresi G, Fini M, Cigada A. (2003) Mechanical and histomorphometric evaluations of titanium implants with different surface treatment inserted in sheep cortical bone. *Biomaterials* **24**: 1583.
57. Giavaresi G, Fini M, Cigada A, Chiesa R, Rondelli G, Rimondini L, Aldini NN, Martini L, Giardino R. (2003) Histomorphometric and microhardness assessments of sheep cortical bone surrounding titanium implants with different surface treatments. *J. Biomed. Mater. Res. A* **67**: 112.
58. Son WW, Zhu X, Shin HI, Ong JL, Kim KH. (2003) In vivo histological response to anodized and anodized/hydrothermally treated titanium implants. *J. Biomed. Mater. Res. B Appl. Biomater.* **66B**: 520.
59. Ishizawa H, Fujino M, and Ogino M. (1997) Histomorphometric evaluation of the thin hydroxyapatite layer formed through anodization followed by hydrothermal treatment. *J. Biomed. Mater. Res.* **35**: 199.
60. Sul YT. (2003) The significance of the surface properties of oxidized titanium to the bone response: special emphasis on potential biochemical bonding of oxidized titanium implant. *Biomaterials* **24**: 3893.
61. Feng B, Wang J, Yang BC, Qu SX, Zhang XD. (2003) Characterization of surface oxide films on titanium and adhesion of osteoblast. *Biomaterials* **24**: 4664.
62. Boyan BD, Batzer R, Kiesewetter K, Lie Y, Cochran DL, Szmuckler-Moncler S, Dean DD, Schwartz Z. (1998) Titanium surface roughness alters responsiveness of MG63 osteoblastic-like cells to 1α,25-$(OH)_2D_3$. *J. Biomed. Mater. Res.* **39**: 77.
63. Karlsson M, Palsgard E, Wilshaw PR, Silvio LD. (2003) Initial in vitro interaction of osteoblasts with nano-porous alumina. *Biomaterials* **24**: 3039.
64. Webster TJ, Ergun C, Doremus RH, Siegel RW, and Bizios R. (2001) Enhanced osteoclast-like cell functions on nanophase ceramics. *Biomaterials* **22**: 1327.
65. Dunn DS, Raghaven S, Volz RG. (1994) Ciprofloxacin attachment to porous coated titanium surfaces. *J. Appl. Biomater.* **5**: 325.
66. Varkey M, Gittens SA, Uludag H. (2004) Growth factor delivery for bone tissue repair: an update. *Expert Opin. Drug Deliv.* **1**: 19.

Chapter 4

Bio-inspired Carbon Nano-structures: Orthopedic Applications

Dongwoo Khang

1. Fundamentals of Protein Adsorption and Surface Properties

Surface interactions between a protein and a solid surface are of paramount importance in tissue engineering as well as biophysics. This is because surface interactions drive protein adsorption and eventually lead to subsequent cellular interactions (Fig. 1) on surfaces.[1] Generally, the protein adsorption process depends both on the physical properties of the surface and structure of the protein.[2,3]

For these reasons, the collective properties of both the protein and material surfaces should be extensively analyzed to improve our understanding of how to increase implant biocompatibility. Surface properties such as chemistry, hydrophilicity, hydrophobicity, roughness, and surface energy have been shown to affect the adsorption of fibronectin, and vitronectin on solid surfaces.[4,8] For example, vitronectin, fibronectin and albumin adsorption increased on hydrophilic surfaces with micron/nano surface roughness or high surface energies.[6,7] Since proteins mediate the adhesion of specific anchorage-dependent cells like osteoblasts and endothelial cells on substrates, the adsorption of vitronectin, laminin and fibronectin on polystyrene subsequently enhances the adhesion of osteoblasts, fibroblasts, and endothelial cells.[8,9] These studies provide evidence that the adsorption of specific proteins enhances subsequent cell adhesion on materials surfaces.

In the same manner, protein adsorption mechanisms are also very important for understanding the success or failure of implant

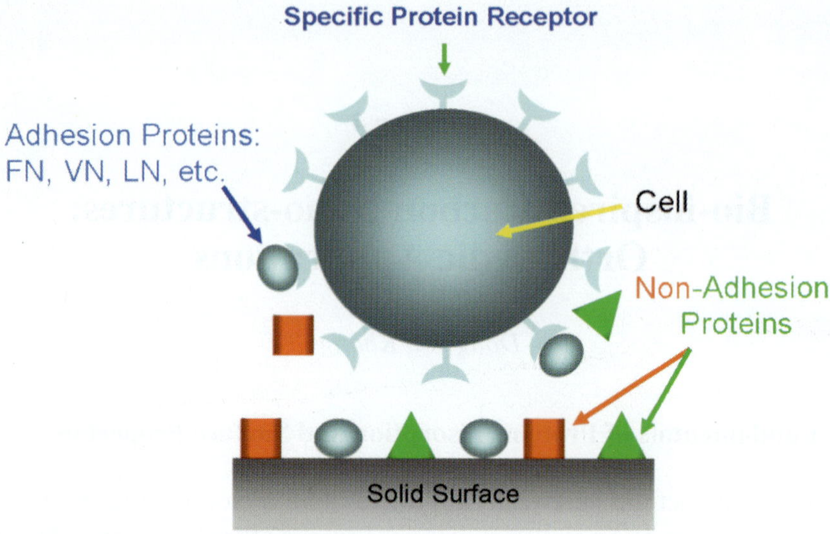

Figure 1. Cell interactions with specific proteins in extracellular fluids: the receptor proteins recognize and cause the cell to adhere to solid substrates. FN, VN and LN represent fibronectin, vitronectin and laminin, respectively.

surfaces in orthopedics. For example, nano-structured surfaces induce high biocompatibility than conventional implant surfaces (such as titanium, gold, amalgams and silicon).[10-12] However, the fundamental understanding of the high cytocompatibility of cells on various nanophase materials and composites has not been clearly elucidated to date, though it is believed that the unique surface properties of nanophase materials can enhance protein adsorption.[10,11,33]

To understand the suggested issues, several investigation techniques for characterizing surfaces are essential as well as basic information of protein and cells interactions. For this reason, this section will discusses about the information of one major cell adhesion protein (fibronectin: FN), functions of bone forming cells (osteoblasts: OB), carbon nanotubes as a source of implant nano surface roughness, characterization of surface roughness via atomic force microscopy (AFM) and lastly a discussion on general surface chemistry/surface energy to analyze the mechanisms of greater protein and enhanced cell adhesion on carbon nano-structured surfaces.

1.1. Adhesion Protein

It is believed that fibronectin mediates anchorage dependent cells adhesion.[46] Fibronectin has molecular weight of around 270kDa and is involved in many cellular processes, including tissue repair, embryogenesis (the process of forming and developing of an embryo), blood clotting, and cell migration/adhesion (Fig. 2).[46] There are several isoforms of fibronectin that are the product of a single gene. The structure of these isoforms are composed of three types of repeated internal regions called I, II and III which exhibit different lengths and the presence or absence of disulfide (negatively-charged ion) bonds. The most abundant module in fibronectin is Type III, which contains the Arg-Gly-Asp (RGD) tri-peptide receptor cell recognition sequence along with the binding sites for other cell membrane integrins (Fig. 2).

1.2. Polar and Apolar Properties of Proteins

Protein molecules have both apolar and polar parts.[25] Such properties are important for electrostatic interactions with charged surfaces and hydrophobic and hydrophilic interactions between proteins and surfaces. In aqueous environments, the apolar residues tend to be buried in the interior of the molecules and shielded from water. However, if other interactions are participating, apolar parts are exposed on the surface of the folded protein structures.

The attractive van der Waals force is a major source of apolar energy between two interfaces.[24] This force arises from fluctuations of atomic dipoles and the polarizability of constituent atoms within the given materials. Though the van der Waals force is not strong like electrostatic or solvation forces in liquids, it is always present between two surfaces, regardless of their size. Though van der Waals forces alone determine domain interactions for non-polar wetting films or surfaces, polar energy originates from electrostatic forces between charges, dipoles, quadrupoles, etc.[24] Coulomb effects are largely dependent on the distribution of charged residues.[25] Also, like van der Waals attractive forces, exactly calculating this energy between two interfaces is very complicated, especially in arbitrary nano-roughness surfaces or nano-composite surfaces.

For relatively small proteins, such as lysozymes, ribonucleases and cytochromes having molar mass about of 1.5kDa, apolar atoms occupy about 40-50% of the surface area accessible to the aqueous environment. For larger proteins like fibronectin, the polar fraction of the surface is higher than in small proteins.[25]

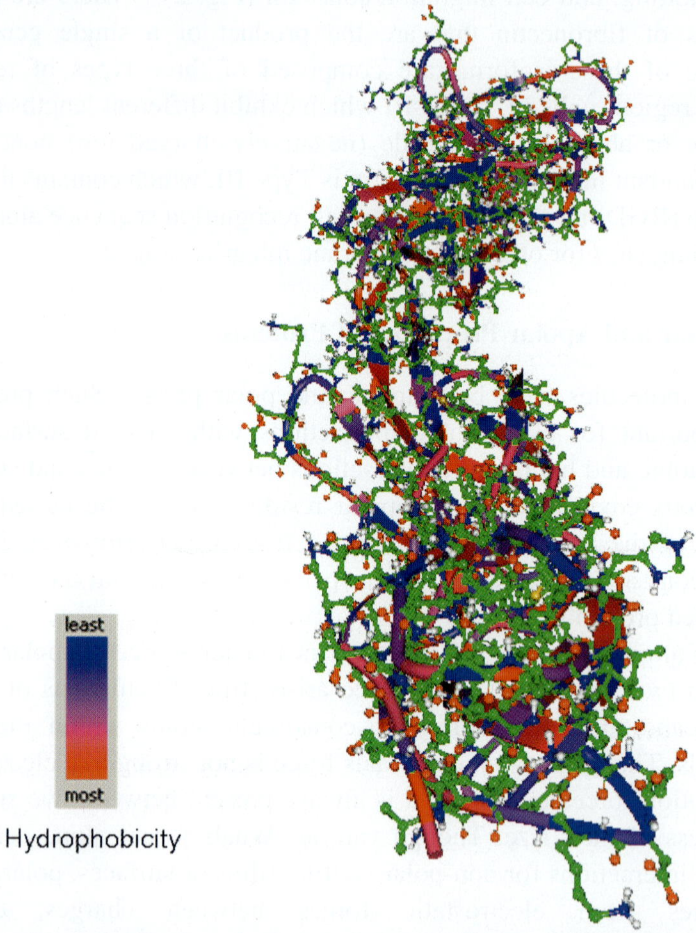

Figure 2. Atomic and ribbon chains of human fibronectin (drawn with molecular biology toolkit: MBT software): Inset shows hydrophilic parts colored blue while hydrophobic parts colored red. Middle parts of fibronectin show type III modules and RGD is abundant in type III modules. For more detail, see dimer and RGD in Fig. 3.

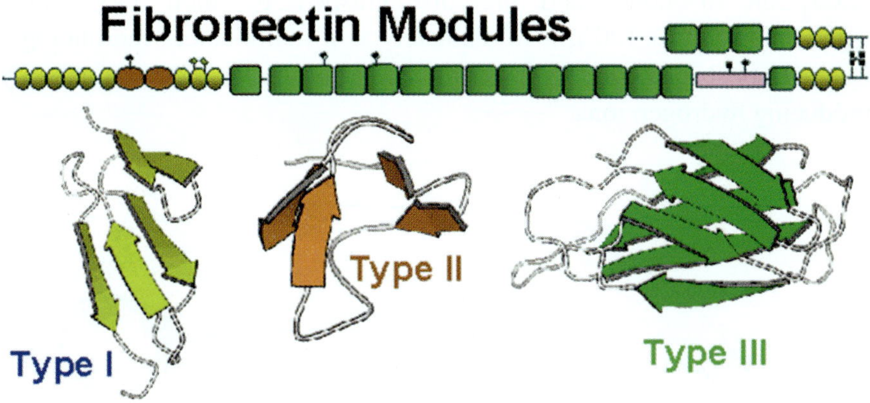

Figure 3. Representation of modules of FN: FN is composed of type I, II and III. A dimer of two identical subunits is covalently linked by a pair of disulfide bonds at type I. RGD sequences are found in type II and III. The image adopted from http://home.comcast.net/~kennethingham/newsite/index.htm. For more detail, see[46].

1.3. Osteoblasts

For bone formation, calcium phosphate crystals (CaP) are important factor for determining oseeo-integration surrounding bone tissues.[19,28] Bone forming cell (osteoblast: OB) can generate such CaP crystals if certain growth factors are regulated in growth media. Interestingly, recent results have shown that bone formation on nano-implant surfaces have shown greater responses than conventional implant surface. Generally, OB comes from mesenchymal stem cells (Fig. 4) and different growth factors determine the differentiation of stem cells into OBs. There are three types of bone cells: OBs, osteocytes and osteoclasts. It is well established that osteoblasts contribute new bone synthesis with osteocytes (mature osteoblasts).[26] Osteocytes regulate new bone formation by modulating osteoblast function through the secretion of growth factors. These growth factors mediate the differentiation of osteoblasts from immature, non-calcium depositing cells into mature osteoblasts that deposited calcium-containing minerals into the extracellar matrix of bone.[26] Osteoclasts are primarily responsible for the absorption of bone, and are distinguished by their large sizes (specifically up to 100 μm in diameter) as a multinuclear morphology. Osteoclasts absorb bone by lowering the pH of the local environment by producing hydrogen ions.[26]

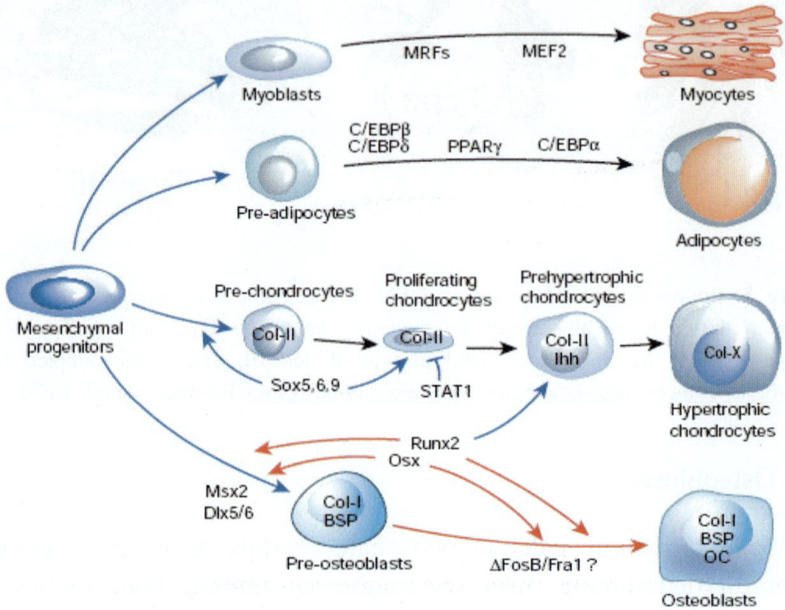

Figure 4. Differentiation of mesenchymal progenitors: mesenchymal progenitor or stem cells differentiated to OBs by specific growth factors (Msx2 and Dix5/6 and ΔFosB/Fra1: see[38] for detail). Image was adopted from[26].

1.4. Carbon Nanotubes and Carbon Nanotube Composites

Due to their low weight/high strength ratio, high conductivity, and ability to mimic the dimensions of constituent components of bone, such as hydroxyapatite and collagen, carbon nanotubes (CNTs) are intriguing formulations for orthopedic applications.[11-12,20-23] CNTs are cylindrical carbon molecules with properties that can be potentially useful in extremely small scale electronic, mechanical and biomedical applications.[27,30] There are two main types of nanotubes: single-walled carbon nanotubes (swCNTs) and multi-walled nanotubes (mwCNTs).

All types of CNTs are composed entirely of sp^2 bonds and sp^2 bonding structures that provide their unique mechanical and electrical properties.[27]

Many of the outstanding properties can be best exploited by incorporating CNTs into some form of matrix.[30-32] In many cases, these composite materials have employed polymer matrices. For biomedical applications, FDA approved polymers are commonly utilized in the human body. A commonly used method for preparing CNT/polymer composites has involved mixing dispersed CNTs with a solution of a particular polymer and then evaporating the solvent in a controlled way. Polycarbonate urethane (PCU) is a thermoplastic polymer that has been used as a matrix for nanotube composites (Fig. 5). To make composites with homogenous nanometer roughness, highly dispersed CNT composites are required. PCU also has a very high melting temperature (200°C) and is non-degradable because it does not react with oxygen. Thus, it is widely used as an implant material in various surgeries because of these suggested advantages.[14,21,41]

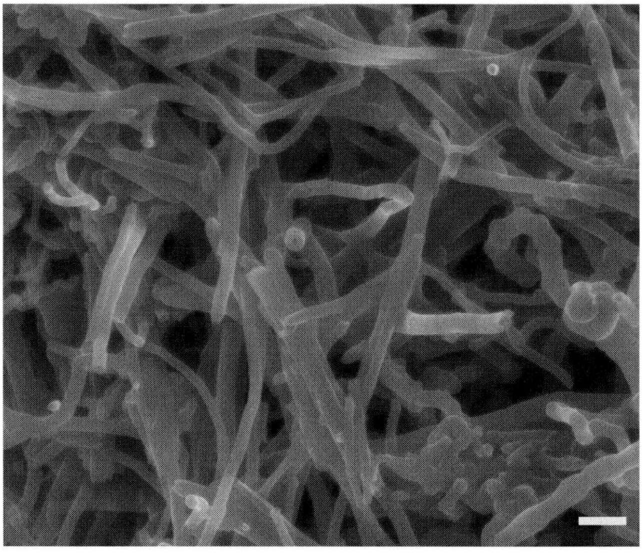

Figure 5. CNF composites: FESEM (Field Emission Scanning Electron Microscope; bar is 100nm) image shows that the CNFs are completely coated by the PCU.

1.5. Cytocompatibility of Carbon Nanotube Composites

Biocompatible materials are defined as materials that do not induce an acute or chronic inflammation response and do not prevent the proper formation of surrounding tissue on an implant.[2] As a such promising biocompatible materials, CNTs have generated a large amount of interest for a number of applications including serving as delivery vehicles for biological molecules, proteins, growth factors, cytokines and pharmaceutical agents.[15-18] Previous reports have demonstrated increased cell adhesion, viability and enhanced deposition of calcium by osteoblasts on CNT based materials placed in polymer composites.[20,28,23,21,22] In attempt to understand why, recent results showed enhanced FN adsorption on CNT/PCU composites.[47] Another advantage of using CNT composites is the ability to control the amount of nano-roughness via different weight ratios of CNTs in PCU that can control the surface energy important factor for controlling biological activities.[47]

1.6. Analysis of Nano-surface Roughness

These CNT composites of various nanometer surface roughness and surface energy have been helpful in understanding fundamental properties of CNTs that increase osteoblasts functions. The most common tool for investigating surface roughness is atomic force microscopy (AFM). AFM has a resolution of several angstrom in both lateral and vertical scanning ranges. The advantage of AFM is that it can be used as a probe for investigating protein interaction on nano-featured surfaces.[43,45] Since many protein sizes are comparable to features of nano surfaces, attached biological substances (such as DNA, peptides and proteins) on AFM tips can be utilized as probe for biological, nano-scale interactions on various nano surfaces (Fig. 6).[17,45] In addition, AFM can be used as a tool for measuring surface roughness and surface area.[33,34] Since nano-scale roughness requires extremely high resolution, the AFM tip is the most suitable probe compared to any other scanning tool. Appropriate resolution of AFM will give surface topography information as well as surface roughness; those properties are important for analyzing protein adsorption on nano-structured surfaces.[33-35]

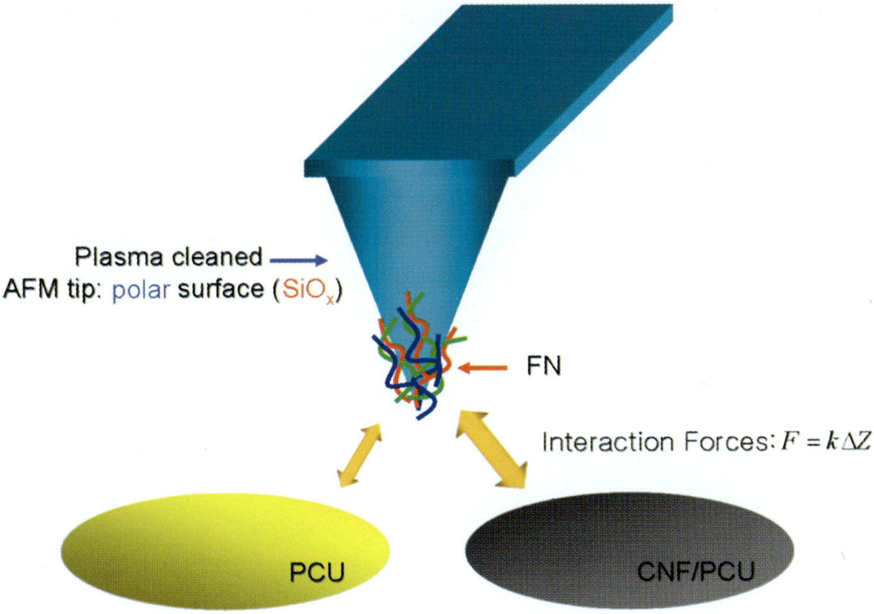

Figure 6. FN adsorbed AFM tip-substrate interactions: plasma cleaned AFM tips (bio-active surface) have been coated with FN to observe its interaction on various nano-roughness surfaces (bio-polymers and CNTs). For interaction forces, k is spring constant for describing order of intrinsic bonding between FN and nano-composite materials. ΔZ represents force affected distance between FN and CNT composite surfaces.

1.7. Role of Nano-surface Energy

Surface energy, determined by complex molecular interactions, is considered to be an important factor for determining protein adsorption or cell adhesion.[42] This is because the polar and non-polar parts of amino acids in protein are selectively interacting with contacted surfaces.[2] In addition, water contact angles, those have polar and non-polar tensions, are easily measured by a contact angle analyzer.[33] For this reason, understanding of contact angles are corresponds to understand of protein interaction with various surfaces as well as providing important information of nano-surface properties on surfaces (Fig. 7). Since hydrophicity and hydrophobicity (usually bigger than 90° of contact angle) are closely related with protein adsorption and their correlations are certainly affecting subsequent cell adhesion, understanding of these properties are directly related with a fundamental understanding of protein and cell responses on surfaces.[24,47] Importantly, nano-surface roughness also can alter both surface energy/contact angles and these altered surface properties can affect protein adsorption and eventually change subsequent cell adhesion. However, quantified investigations of surface energy coupled with nanoscale surface roughness and their relation to protein adsorption/cell adhesion are not clear.[11, 33-35]

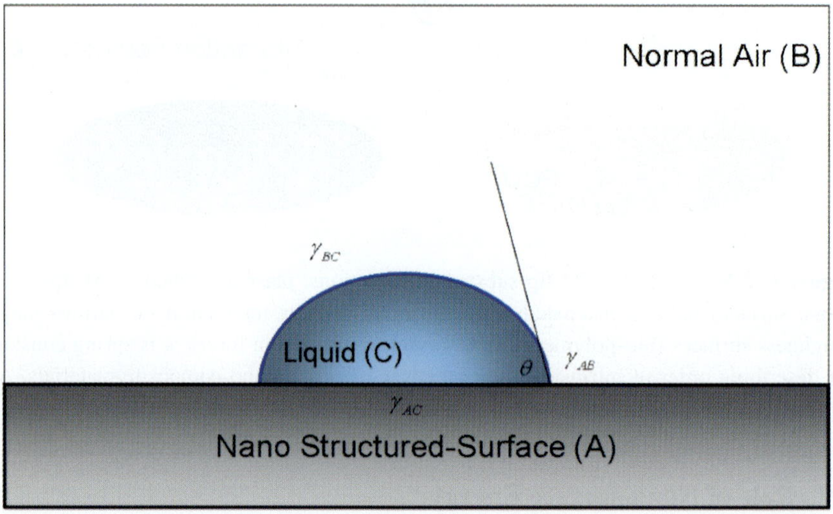

Figure 7. Intermediate partial wetting: surface tension between nano-structured surfaces (A) and liquid (C) determines the contact angle (theta) in ambient condition (B). γ is surface tension between two interacting materials.

1.8. Detecting Protein Adsorption

There are several methods for detecting protein adsorption such as: X-ray photon electron spectroscopy, Raman spectroscopy, fluorescence, infrared spectroscopy, ELISA (Enzyme-Linked Immunosorbent Assay) and surface plasmon resonance methods. In ELISA experiments, FN is directly linked with specific antibodies in aqueous environments; such antibodies are then detected by a direct fluorescence photon detector (Fig. 8). For ELISA tests, antibodies were utilized to produce a fluorescence signal. These antibodies were linked with specific enzymes which react with chromogenic materials (Fig. 8).

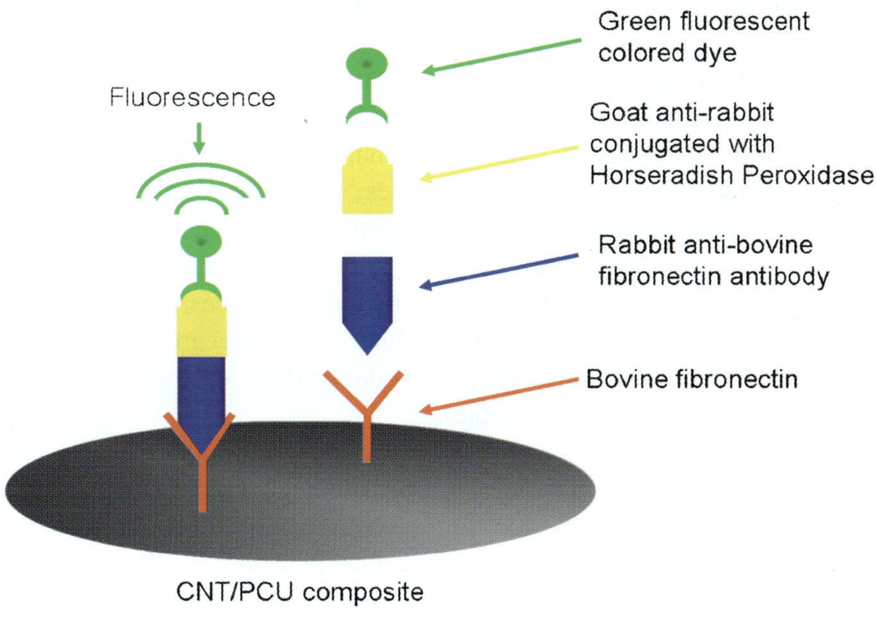

Figure 8. ELISA-antibody reaction with fibronectin on carbon nanotube composite surfaces (See text for details).

2. Protein Assisted Osteoblast Adhesion on Nanophase Materials

Extensive studies reveal that the adhesion of proteins like FN, VN, LN and collagen are strongly related with cell adhesion and indeed, greater protein adsorption has been found on nano-structured materials compared to conventional smooth implant surfaces.[4,10-12,21-23] The most plausible mechanism for this occurrence is that nanoscale roughness or nanoscale surface topography may affect surface energies on nano structured surfaces and eventually lead to more protein adsorption.[21,33,34] Experimental results show that FN adsorption was higher on nano-structured surfaces compared to other proteins and thus, much more effort should be focused on the properties of these nano surfaces and how they can control proteins (which have the RGD sequence adsorption).[46] Recent studies also have shown enhanced FN adsorption on CNT composites compared to smooth polymer surfaces.[47]

From the surface property aspect, arbitrary nano-structured surfaces have shown incremental increases in surface energy through increasing nano-surface roughness.[44,48] However, nano-pillar structures (vertical tube structures) have shown decreases in surface energy.[40,44] An important point is that all protein adsorption is increased on nano-structured surfaces, regardless of hydrophilic (arbitrary nano-structures) and hydrophobic (pillar or tube nano-structures) surfaces. This is can be explained by the fact that surface roughness is another important factor for controlling protein adsorption bedsides surface chemistry (surface energy: hydrophilic or hydrophobic).

In this section, we will look over previous study which has specifically correlated OB adhesion on various CNT composite surface roughnesses. Also, FN adhesion force measurements will be discussed to explain why OBs have been to adhere more on nano-structured surfaces than on smooth bio-polymer surfaces. Also, micro-aligned patterns of CNTs are discussed because they can control the morphology of adherent cells and thus shows direct evidence of selective responses of bone cells.

2.1. Osteoblast Functions on Carbon Nanotube Composite Materials

Osteoblast adhesion tests were performed on CNT composite materials.[21,22] The fabrication techniques used in those studies were used to increase the amount of CNTs in a polymer matrix. Interestingly, results showed that osteoblast adhesion increased with the incremental weight percentage increase of CNTs in PCU (Fig. 9). Because the amount CNTs in PCU directly corresponds to nano-surface roughness, increased nano-surface roughness induces greater adhesion of OBs. Figure 9a shows high cytocompatibility of bone cells on CNTs in PCU with greater nano-surface roughness.

Alternatively, smooth muscle cells and fibroblasts show different adhesion tendency on CNTs in PCU compared to osteoblasts (Figure 9). In short, fibroblast adhesion on CNT composites shows decreased adhesion of fibroblast compared to control or nano-featured surfaces created by CNT alone. Recent studies revealed that surface energy and surface roughness are systematically affected to adsorption of protein and anchorage cell adhesions like osteoblasts.[47]

Most importantly, previous studies have shown superior cytocompatibility for smaller diameters of CNTs that leads more osseo-integration, compare to conventional dimension of CNTs (Fig. 10). Because of low diameter of CNT are corresponds to small roughness which gives small surface energy, results also provided the evidence that initial surface properties are determines the long term functions of bone cells as well as affect to short term adhesion.

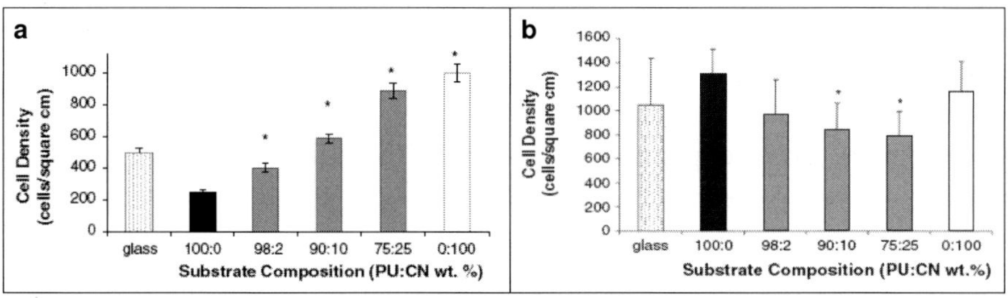

Figure 9. (a) Increased OB adhesion density on CNTs composites. (b) Decreased fibroblasts on CNTs composites. Values are Mean +/– SEM; n = 3; *p<0.1 Compared to 100:0 (PCU: CNT) wt %. See[21] for more detail.

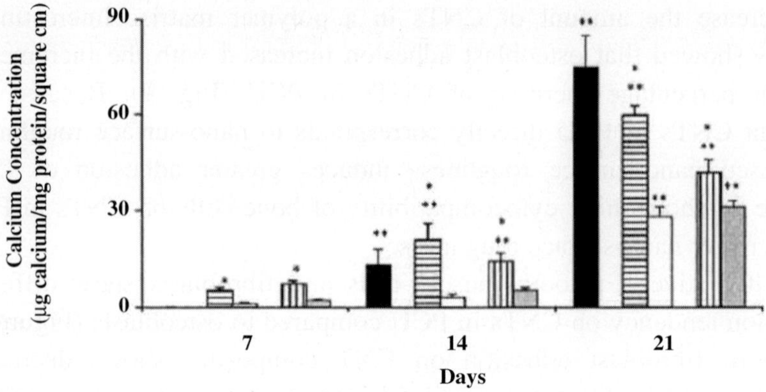

Figure 10. Enhanced deposition of calcium on smaller dimensioned carbon nanofibers. Osteoblasts in DMEM (supplemented with 10% FBS, 50 μg/ml L-ascorbate, 10mM β-glycerophosphate, 1% penicillin streptomycin, and 1.5% geneticin) were cultured on the following substrates: ■ borosilicate glass (reference substrate), ⊟ PR-1 AG (nanophase: 100 nm diameter with a pyrolytic outer core), □ PR-19 AG (conventional: 200 nm diameter with a pyrolytic outer core), ◫ PR-24 PS (nanophase: 60 nm diameter without a pyrolytic outer core), and ▩ PR-23 PS (conventional: 125 nm diameter without a pyrolytic outer core). Values are mean +/- SEM; n = 3; *p < 0.01 (compared to respective conventional outer layer carbon fiber compacts); **p < 0.01 (compared to respective substrates at 7 days). See[28] for more detail.

2.2. Fibronectin Attached AFM Tip Interactions on Carbon Nanotube Composite Surfaces

For more fundamental understanding, protein level investigation is essential since specific protein (like FN, VN) have been known to mediate OB adhesion. To examine any differences in FN adsorption that occurred on CNT composites and soft bio-polymers (like PCU), interactions force experiments between FN attached AFM tips and various surface roughness were conducted.[43,45] FNs were the focus of this investigation since this protein mediates OB adhesion.[46] Reference AFM tips (without any FN) showed constant forces with all regions of the surfaces of both CNT and PCU (Fig. 11).

Specifically, adhesion forces were around 5nN for both CNT composite surfaces and PCU with uncoated tips. This means that the conventional AFM tip (Si-Ox) had no preferential interactions on the nano-structured polymer compared to the soft polymer in ambient

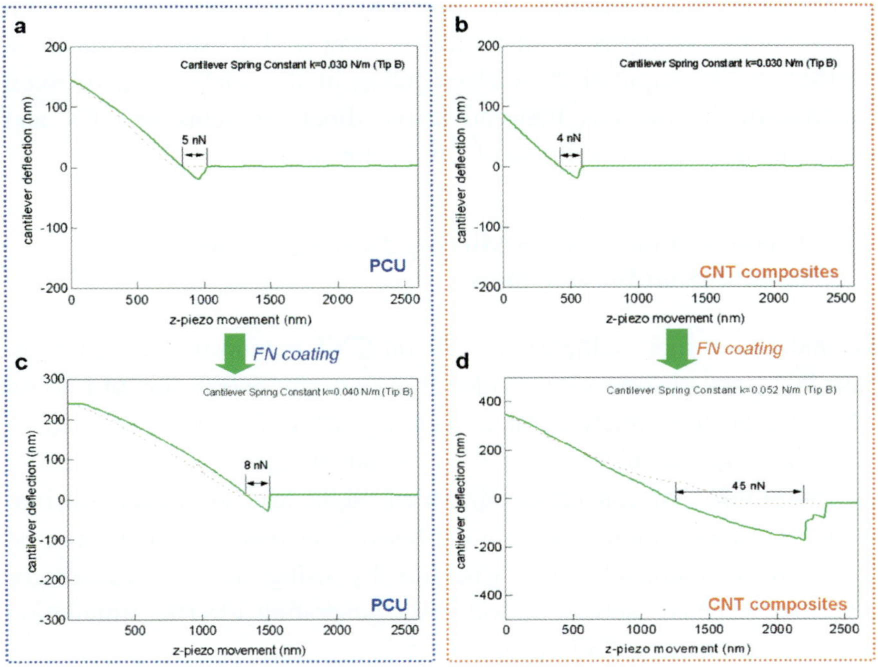

Figure 11. (a) AFM tip interaction (Tip Without FN) on PCU. (b) AFM tip interaction (Tip Without FN) on CNT composite surfaces. (c) FN coated AFM tip interaction on PCU. (d) FN coated AFM tip interaction on CNT composite surface.

conditions (humidity of 20-30% at room temperature ~300K. See[41] for detail).

Interesting results (Fig. 11) were also obtained when examining the interactions between FN adsorbed AFM tips on PCU and CNT composite surfaces. Specifically, the adhesion force of FN attached AFM tips were around 15nN (Fig. 11) for PCU but were 45nN for CNT composites (Fig. 11). The observed force range distance also shows an interesting fact: long range interactions (Figure 11). Since van der Waals force range is just a few ~Å and unfolding of domains in FN are less than a hundred nanometers, observed long range interactions (more than 1 μm) may results from electrostatic forces from FN and nano structured surfaces (or high energies).[24,43,45] This suggests that coulomb interactions (mono, dipoles, quadrupoles, etc.) of FN may be strongly correlated with increased nano-roughness on surfaces, compared to smooth surfaces. Further studies required the understanding of the relationship between electrostatic interactions between heavy dipole proteins like FN and greater nano-surface roughness of CNT composites.

2.3. Osteoblast Functions on Micro-patterning of Carbon Nanotubes on Bio-polymers

To understand more adhesion of OB on CNT composites compared to base PCU, and observe clear evidence of preferred interaction of FNs on CNT composites, micro-aligned pattering of CNT has developed in recently.[41] Aligned patterns have several advantages: First, it can affect the morphology of cell adhesion, which might lead to aligned calcium minerals similar to long bones in the body.[19] Second, advantages can be found in such aligned nano-structures by using them as censer for detecting selective adhesion, and even generating electric stimulation along the conducting CNTs patterns.[18,20,41]

Because CNTs require toxic solvents to reacts with solid surfaces, previous known protocols for fabricating aligned patterns cannot be applied using bio-polymers.[36,37] This is because biopolymers are easily dissolved in such solvents. For this reason, new techniques have been recently developed for patterning of nano-particles (e.g., nanotubes, nanoparticles, nanospheres, etc.) on widely used FDA approved polymers for clinical and direct use for *in vitro* applications.[41]

This novel technique does not require any toxic solvents to react CNTs on the substrate but utilizes simply the bonding forces between CNTs and polymer surfaces employing a grid method (Fig. 12).

SEM images of these structures show highly aligned CNF arrays successfully imprinted onto PCU by the novel grid alignment method (Fig. 12). Aligned CNF arrays were arranged 30μm apart to control osteoblast alignment (see Fig. 12). The density of imbedded CNFs was controlled by the amount of carbon nanofibers in solution in the Au grid. AFM cross sectional height data showed a very thick CNF density which allows two totally different materials to interact (Fig. 12).

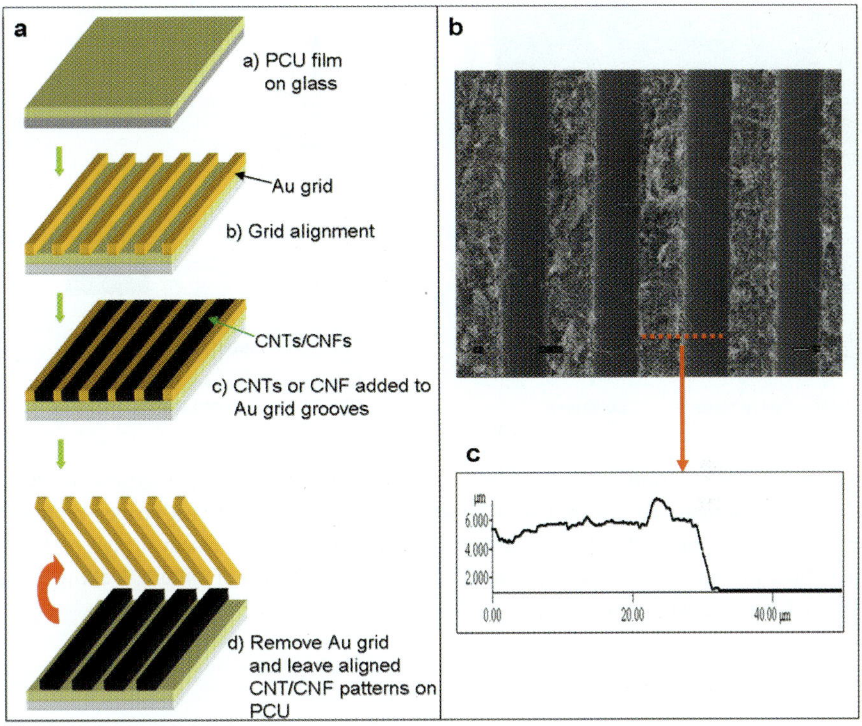

Figure 12. (a) Schematic diagram of aligned CNTs/CNFs arrays on PCU. (b) SEM image (500X, red bar is 60μm) of localized higher densities of CNF arrays on PCU. (c) Cross-sectional height data: average height of aligned patterns of CNF is around 5 μm and it shows greater thickness of CNFs.

Importantly, OB adhesion results provided the evidence that human OB selectively adhered on CNT patterns compared to PCU arrays (Figure 13). Specifically, more than 80% of the OB adhered on CNTs or CNFs arrays but less than 20% on the PCU.[41] As discussed in the previous section, this might be due to higher interactions (through increased surface energy) of FN on greater nano-roughness surfaces. This suggests that electrical stimulation can be generated along the arrays of CNT after the selective adhesion of OB on non-conductive bio-polymers.

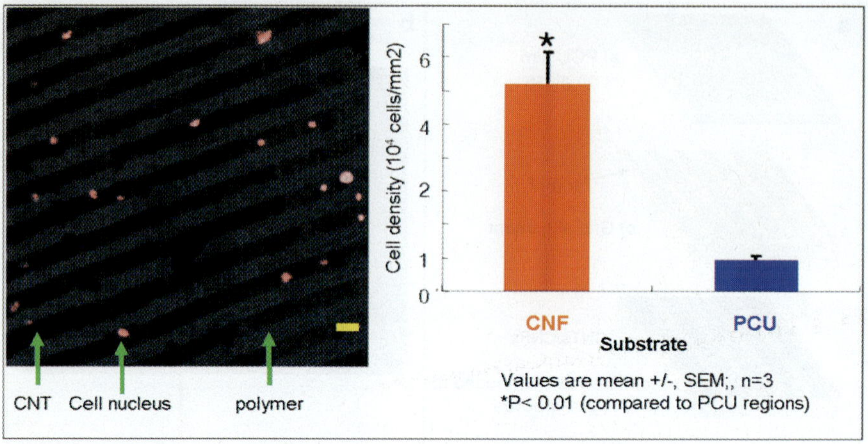

Figure 13. Optical fluorescence images of OB on aligned CNF/CNT arrays on PCU: Majority of human OB adhered on CNFs/CNTs, not on PCU. Black stripes represent arrays of CNTs or CNFs. Bright stripes (relative to black) represent arrays of PCU. Red objects represents adherent human OB nucleus after 2 days of culture. Yellow bar is 30 μm. For more detail, see[63].

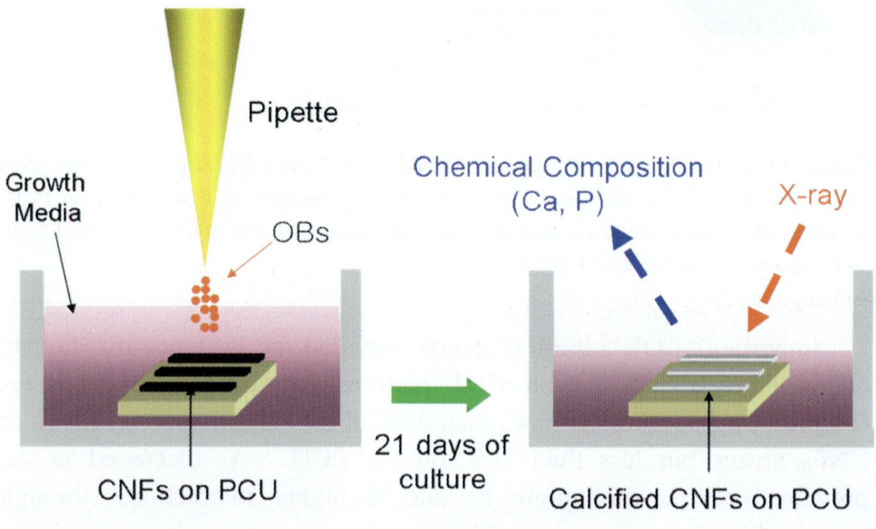

Figure 14. Detection of calcium phosphate-crystals: osteoblasts cultured with confluent seeding density (60,000 cells/cm^2). Differentiation of osteoblast was controlled by growth factors (β-glycerophosphate and l-ascorbic acid) to generate calcium phosphate crystals. After 21 days, aligned calcium phosphate signals were detected by EDX.

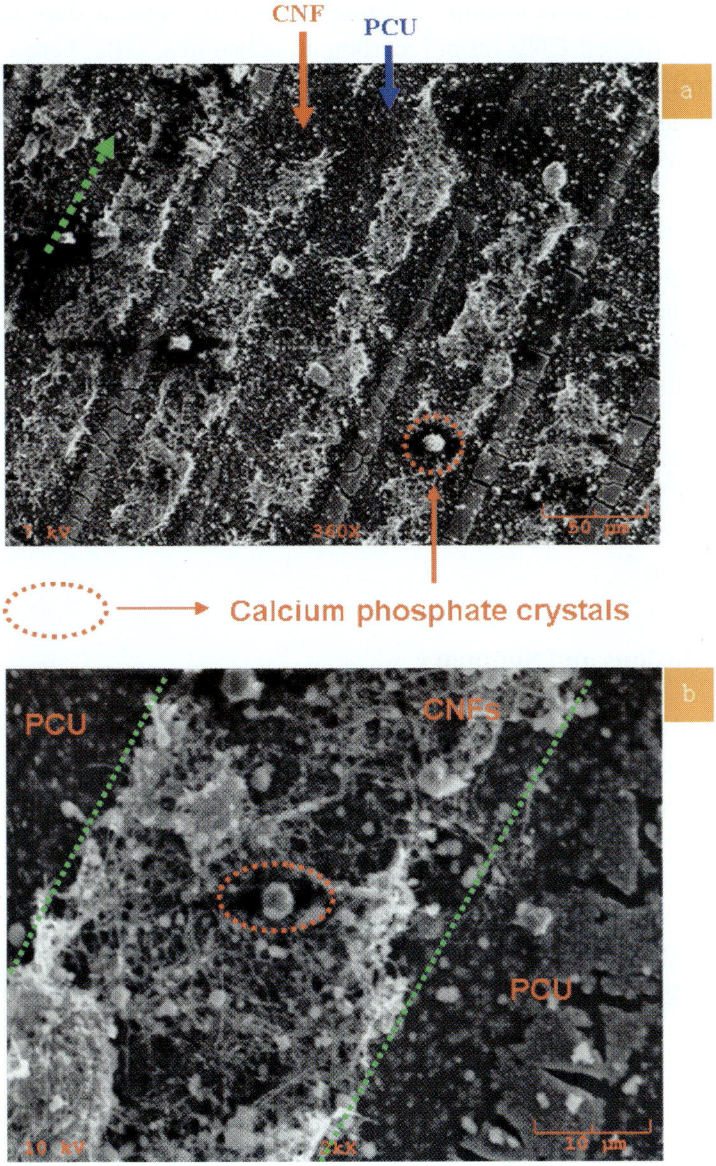

Figure 15. Deposition of CaP crystals: SEM image shows more deposition of CaP crystals in CNFs than PCU (a and b). OB were cultured for 21 days. Bars are 50 μm (a) and 10 μm (b).

In addition, to determine calcium phosphate mineral deposition on the micro-aligned CNF on polycarbonate substrates, OBs were cultured with confluent seeding density for 21 days. After 21 days of OB culture, directed deposition of calcium phosphate (CaP) minerals was observed on arrays of CNF compared to PCU, using SEM and EDS (Figs. 14 and 15). Thus, the results of this study demonstrate the ability to mimic the alignment of hydroxyapatite (calcium phosphate ceramic: HA) in bone on micro-patterned CNFs on PCU.

This result was expected since directed adhesion of OBs occurred along regions of CNF compared with PCU. Thus, it could be expected that CaP minerals would be deposited along these same regions. This result is significant as it suggests that the micro alignment of CaP crystals that occurs naturally in long bones of the body can be mimicked by aligning CNFs on PCU. Such alignment can result in directed OB adhesion and subsequent CaP mineral deposition on the CNF regions.[41]

3. Conclusions and Summary

As described here, bio-inspired carbon nanotube structures have many advantages and indeed show promising cytocompatibility for future nano-biotechnology applications. Though present studies focus on cell or protein responses on carbon nanostructured surfaces, more studies on nano-surface properties towards controlling molecular/atomic level will elucidate strong interactions of specific proteins and cells on nano-structured surface. Future studies need to emphasize in vivo experiments using suggested materials and on applying electrical stimulation for promoting the adsorption/adhesion of biological substances to enhance the biocompatibility of nano-structured materials.

Bibliography

1. Ratner B D. (1996) *Biomaterials Sciences* Elsevier Science, New York, NY.
2. Dee K C, Puleo D A and Bizios R. (2002) *An Introduction to Tissue-Biomaterials Interactions* John and Wiley, New Jersey.

3. Luck M. (1998) Analysis of plasma protein adsorption on polymeric nanoparticles with different surface characteristics. *J. Biomed. Mat. Res.* **39**: 478-485.
4. Degasne I. (1999) Effects of roughness, fibronectin and vitronectin on attachment, spreading, proliferation of human osteoblast like cells on titanium surfaces. *Calcified Tissue International* **64**: 499-507.
5. Dalton B A. (1995) Polymer surface chemistry and bone cell migration. *J. Biomat. Sci. Poly.* **8**: 781-799.
6. Lopes M A. (1999) Hydrophobicity, surface tension, and zeta potential measurement of glass–reinforced hydroxyapatite composites. *J. Biomed. Mater. Res.* **45**: 370-375.
7. Horbett TA. (1993) The principles underlying the role of adsorbed plasma proteins in blood interactions with foreign materials. *Cardiovasc. Pathol.* **2**: 137-148.
8. Underwood P and Bennet A. (1989) Comparison of the biological activities of the cell-adhesive proteins vitronectin and fibronectin. *J. Cell Sci.* **93**: 641-649.
9. Thomas CH. (1997) The role of vitronectin in the attachment and spatial distribution of bone derived cells on materials with pattered surface chemistry. *J. Biomed. Mater. Res.* **37**: 81-93.
10. Webster TJ, Schadler LS, Siegel RW, Bizios R. (1999) Mechanism of enhanced osteoblast adhesion on nanophase alumina involve vitronectin. *Tissue Engineering* **7**: 291-302.
11. Webster TJ, Siegel RW, Bizios R. (2000) Specific proteins mediate enhanced osteoblast adhesion on nanophase ceramics. *J. Biomed. Mater. Res.* **51**: 475-483.
12. Webster TJ, Siegel RW, Bizios R. (1999) Osteoblast adhesion on nanophase ceramics. *Biomaterials* **20**: 1221-1227.
13. Silva G A. (2004) Selective differentiation of neural progenitor cells by high-epitope density nanofibers. *Science* **303**: 1352-1354.
14. Thapa A, Webster TJ, Haberstroh KM. (2004) Polymers with nano-dimensional surface features enhance bladder smooth muscle cell adhesion. *Biomaterials* **25**: 53-61.
15. Wang S. (2003) Peptides with selective affinity for carbon nanotubes. *Nature Materials* **7**: 196-200.
16. Barisci J N. (2004) Properties of carbon nanotube fibers spun from DNA- stabilized dispersions. *Advanced Materials* **14**: 133-138.
17. Wong S S. (1998) Covalently functionalized nanotubes as nanometre- sized probes in chemistry and biology. *Nature* **394**: 52-55.
18. Sirdeshmukh R.(2004) Biological functionalization of carbon nanotubes. *Mat. Res. Soc. Symp. Proc.* **823**: w 4.1.1-w 4.1.6.
19. Hartgerink J D. (2001) Self-assembly and mineralization of peptide-amphiphile nanofibers. *Science* **294**: 1684-1688.
20. Supronowicz P R, Ajayan P, Bizios R. (2002) Novel current-conducting composite substrates for exposing osteoblasts to alternating current stimuli. *Journal of Biomedical Material Research* **59**: 499-506.

21. Webster T J, McKenzie J L, Waid MC, Ejiofor J. (2004) Nano-biotechnology: carbon nanofibres as improved neural and orthopedic implants. *Nanotechnology* **15**: 48-54.
22. Price R L, Haberstroh K M, Webster T J. (2003) Selective bone cell adhesion on formulations containing carbon nanofibers. *Biomaterials* **24**: 1877-1887.
23. Price R L, Haberstroh KM, Webster T J. (2004) Improved osteoblast viability in the presence of smaller nanometer dimensioned carbon fibres. *Nanotechnology* **15**: 892-900.
24. Israelachvili J. (1997) *Intermolecular Surface Forces (2nd edition).* Academic Press, New York, NY.
25. Norde W. (2003) Diving forces for protein adsorption at solid surfaces. In: *Biopolymers at Interfaces* (Malmstem M. ed.) Academic Press, New York, NY.
26. Harada S I and Rodan G A. (2002). Control of osteoblast function and regulation of bone mass. *Nature* **423**: 349-355.
27. Smalley RE. (1996) *Carbon Nanotubes: Synthesis, Structure, Properties and Applications* Elsevier Sci, New York, NY.
28. Elias K, Price RL, Webster TJ. (2002) Enhanced fucntion of osteoblasts on nanometer diameter carbon fibers. *Biomaterials* **23**: 3279-3287.
29. McKenzie J L, Shi R, Webster TJ. (2003) Decreased function of astrocytes on carbon nanofibers materials. *Biomaterials* **25**: 1309-1317.
30. Harris P J F. (2004) Carbon nanotube composites. *International Materials Reviews* **49**: 31-43.
31. Sennett M. (2003) Dispersion and alignment of carbon nanotubes in polycarbonate. *Appl. Phys. A* **76**: 111-113.
32. Shaffer M S P and Windle A H. (1999) Fabrication and characterization of carbon nanotube/poly(vinyl alcohol) composites. *Adv. Mater.* **11**: 937-941.
33. Muller B. (2001) Impact of nanometer-scale roughness on contact-angle hysteresis and globulin adsorption. *J. Vac. Sci. Technol. B.* **31**: 1715-1720.
34. Denis FA. (2002) Protein adsorption on model surfaces with controlled nanotopography and chemistry. *Langmuir* **18**: 819-828.
35. Hallab N J. (2001) Evaluation of metallic and polymeric biomaterial surface energy and surface roughness characteristics for directed cell adhesion. *Tissue Engineering* **7**: 55-71.
36. Xia Y and Whitesides G M. (1995) Use of controlled reactive spreading of liquid alkanethiol on the surface of gold to modify the size of features produced by microcontact printing. *J. Am. Chem. Soc.* **117**: 3274-3275.
37. Rao S G. (2003) Nanotube electronics: Large-scale assembly of carbon nanotubes. *Nature* **425**: 36-37.
38. Meitl M A. (2004) Solution casting and transfer printing single-walled carbon nanotube films. *Nano-Letters* **14**: 1643-1647.

39. Falconnet D. (2004) A novel approach to produce protein nanopatterns by combining nanoimprint lithography and molecular self-assembly. *Nano-Letters* **19**: 1909-1914.
40. Kim P. (2005) Fabrication of nanostructures of polyethylene glycol for applications to protein adsorption and cell adhesion. *Nanotechnology* **24**: 2420-2426.
41. Khang D. and Webster TJ. (2006) Selective adhesion and mineral deposition by osteoblasts on carbon nanofiber patterns. *International Journal of Nanomedicine* **1**: 65-72.
42. Schakenraad J M. (1986). The influence of substratum surface free energy on growth and spreading of human fibroblasts in the presence and absence of serum proteins. *Journal of Biomedical Materials Research* **10**: 773-784.
43. Meadow P Y and Walker C. (2005) Force studies of fibronectin adsorption and subsequent cellular adhesion to substrates with well-defined surface chemistries. *Langmuir* **21**: 4096-4107.
44. McHale G. (2004) Topography driven spreading. *Physical Review Letters* **93**: 036102.
45. Oberdorfer Y. (2003) Impact of compatible solutes on the mechanical properties of fibronectin: a single molecule analysis. *PCCP* **5**: 1876-1881.
46. Yamada K M. (1991) Adhesive recognition sequences. *The Journal of Biological Chemistry* **15**: 12809-12812.
47. Khang D and Webster TJ. (2006) The role of nano surface roughness on fibronectin adsorption. *Biomaterials*, in press.
48. Chow T S. (1998) Wetting of rough surfaces. *J. Phys. Condens. Mater.* **10**: 445-451.
49. Nam YS and Park TG. (1996) Porous biodegradable polymeric scaffolds prepared by thermally induced phase separation. *Journal of Biomedical Materials Research* **47**: 17-21.

Chapter 5

Applications of Nanotechnology/Nanomaterials in the Nervous System

Peishan Liu-Snyder

1. Anatomy, Physiology and Molecular Biology of the Nervous System

The human nervous system has two subdivisions which are the central nervous system (CNS) and the peripheral nervous system (PNS). The central nervous system consists of the brain and spinal cord (Fig. 1). They reside within the bony structures which are called the skull for the brain and the vertebrae for the spinal cord. The vertebral columns that enclose the spinal cord divide into five segments of 26 bones. This includes seven cervical vertebrae, twelve thoracic vertebrae, five lumbar vertebrae, one fused sacral vertebrae and one fused coccygeal vertebrae from rostral to caudal. There are two ways to classify the brain based on either embryological origin or function. For the former, the brain further divides into cerebral hemispheres, thalamus, midbrain, pons and cerebellum and medulla oblongata where the brain connects the spinal cord.[1] The spinal cord is the continuity of the brain, which contains large quantities of nerve fibers and neurons and looks like a horse tail. As indicated by its name, the peripheral nervous system resides outside of brain and spinal cord (Fig. 1). It includes both neurons and nerve fibers. The majority of these neurons are located near the spinal cord at ganglia. Nerve fibers extend to sensory structures, glands, blood vessels or muscles.

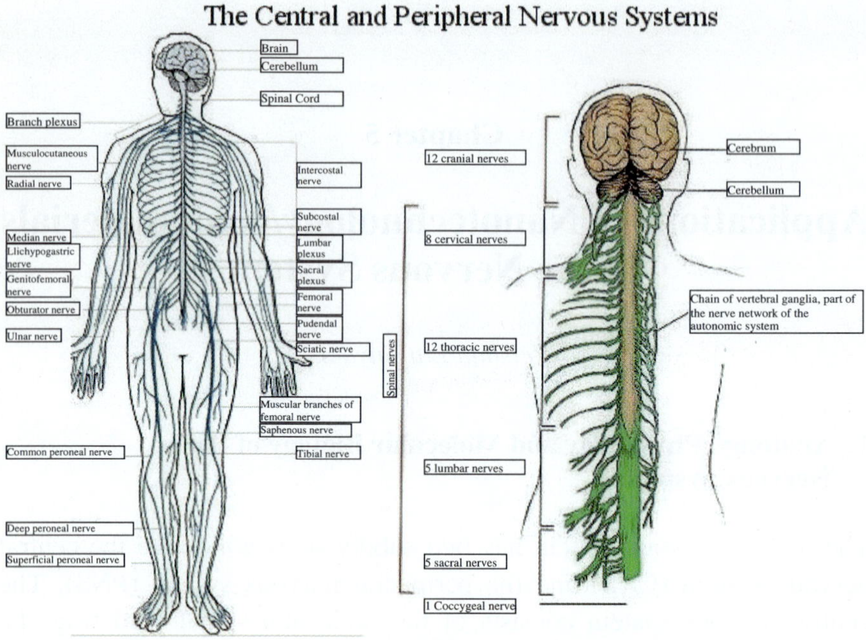

Figure 1. Human nervous system (the central and peripheral nervous systems).

The brain and spinal cord are enfolded by three layers of membranes which are pia matter, arachnoid matter and dura matter (from inside out) embedded with extensive networks of blood vessels which supply the nervous system with sufficient oxygen and glucose. The metabolism of the CNS is very active. The brain weighs five percent of the body mass nevertheless, consumes 20 percent oxygen. Between the pia matter and arachnoid matter, the space is filled with cerebrospinal fluid which not only serves as a cushion but also supports the mass of the brain. The fluid circulates freely and actively within the central canal of spinal cord and ventricles of the brain.[2] The paracellular passage of the molecules to the brain has been tightly regulated by the blood brain barrier (BBB) (Fig. 2A) depending on their size, charge and hydrophobicity. The blood brain barrier forms mainly by the existence of tight junctions (Fig. 2B) between neighboring endothelial cells that line up the blood vessels. Tight junctions form the "narrow zone" of interendothelial clefts and the absence of them are called the "wide zone" (15 ~ 20 nm).[3] But astrocytes and pericytes play an important role in the formation and maintenance of the BBB as well.[4] Only alcohol and few small molecules can freely diffuse through the BBB. Most of molecules that are larger than 400 ~ 500 Dalton need a transporter in order to overcome the barrier.

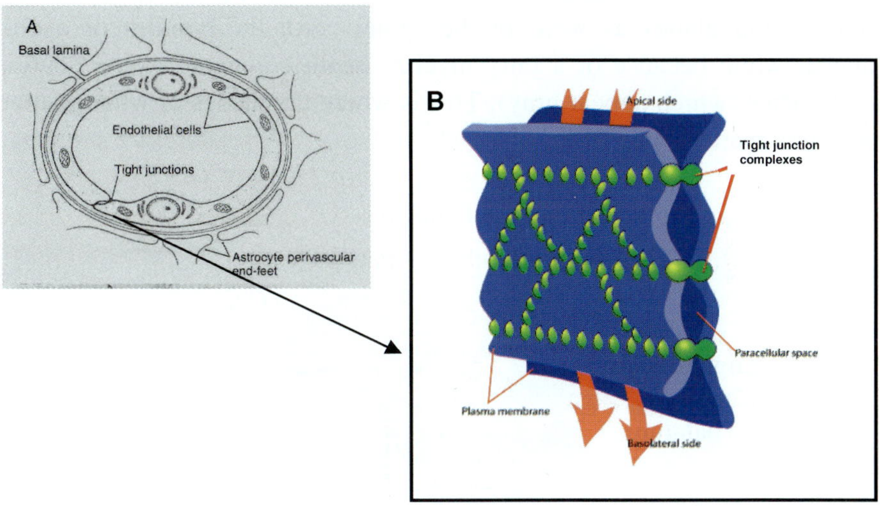

Figure 2. The blood brain barrier (BBB) (A) and tight junction complexes (B) (reprinted from[1]).

As we live in a dynamic environment, our bodies have to be aware of the environment and take appropriate actions to adapt to changes. We achieve this with the help of our nervous system. In the somatic nervous system, the receptors located at sensory structures work as transducers converting different energies from the environment into electrical signals. These electrical signals are picked up by afferent nerve fibers that carry them to the central nervous system. Information can flow to two general directions at this point. One way is to go through simple reflex arcs to motor neurons via afferent fibers to control muscle contraction and the other is to transport to the brain by means of ascending pathways (Fig. 3) in the spinal cord which consist of bundles of nerve fibers. The brain, in most cases, is the place for information analysis and interpretation. Once the decision is made, electrical signals are sent down through descending pathway (Fig. 3) in the spinal cord and leave the spinal cord via efferent nerve fibers to the muscles.[2] As a result, we can voluntarily move our bodies. In this sense, the spinal cord is the connection between brain and the rest of body. Moreover, our autonomic nervous system can unconsciously control smooth muscles, cardiac muscle and glands as well. In the spinal cord, the bundles of axons appear white because of a fatty myelin sheath compared to the neuron cell bodies (which appear gray). This is where the names of white matter and gray matter come from.

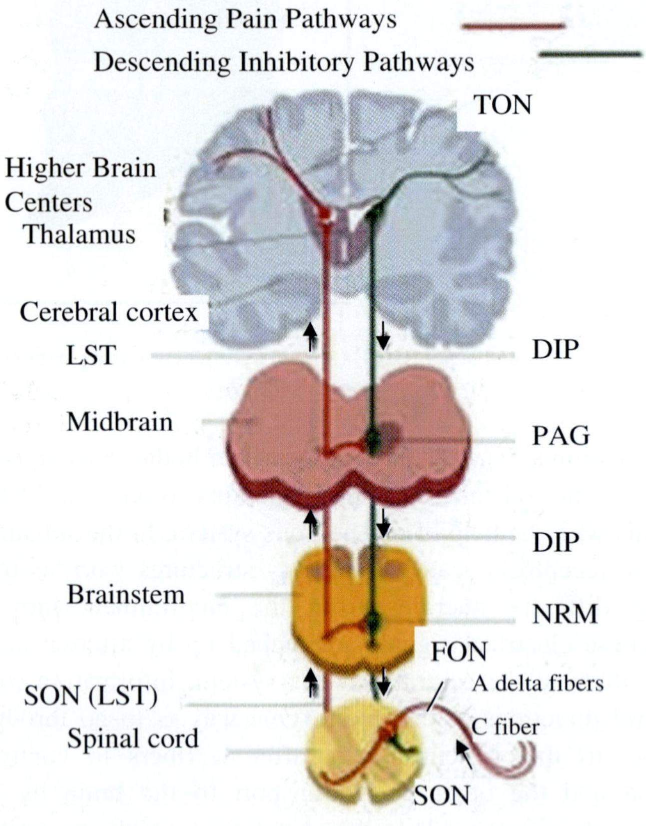

Figure 3. The ascending and descending pathways (reprint from[5]).

Two major classes of cells, neurons and glia (Fig. 4A, B), exist in the nervous system. They play different roles in the nervous system. Glia not only provide structural support for neurons but also regulate neuronal activities.[1] Though glia outnumber neurons, the major functional units of the CNS and PNS are neurons. In the absence of stimuli, the neuron membrane maintains a steady level which is determined by electrochemical gradients of ions mainly K^+, Na^+ and Ca^{2+} across the membrane. In most cases, it is -40 mV to – 90 mV.[6] The chemical gradient is not balanced across the membrane at resting since there are more sodium ions outside and potassium ions inside the cells. Neurons actually consume lots of energy to pump sodium out and potassium in constantly. When sodium ion channels on the membrane open upon stimulation, sodium ions will flow down the chemical gradients. Once membranes become depolarized to a threshold, neurons evoke an action potential which propagates along the nerve fiber in such a way that the information can be transported to other cells nearby and far away. Each neuron has a cell body, dendrites and an axon. The axon and dendrites of neurons form networks with other neurons by making contacts at synapses. Synapses are fluid-filled gaps between the terminal endings of axons or dendrites. The neuromuscular synapses have been used as an example to elucidate how it works.[6]

The axon of a motor neuron swells at the pre-synaptic terminal ending where electron microscopy images have revealed abundant vesicles containing neurotransmitters, in this case, acetylcholine. The post-synaptic terminal ending with a muscle cell lies very close to the pre-synaptic terminal, however, it is separated by synapse cleft. On the surface of post-synaptic membranes there exist the receptors to acetylcholine which are also ion channels. When a nerve impulse conducts down to the pre-synaptic terminal, acetylcholine releases into the synaptic cleft. Once it binds to its receptor, the ion channel opens to sodium ions. Sodium influx depolarizes the post-synaptic membrane which triggers the release of calcium from sarcoplasmic reticulum in the muscle cell. As a result, muscles contract.

Both neurons and glia contain several types.[1] For example, glia in the brain are divided into three classes, oligodendrocytes, astrocytes and

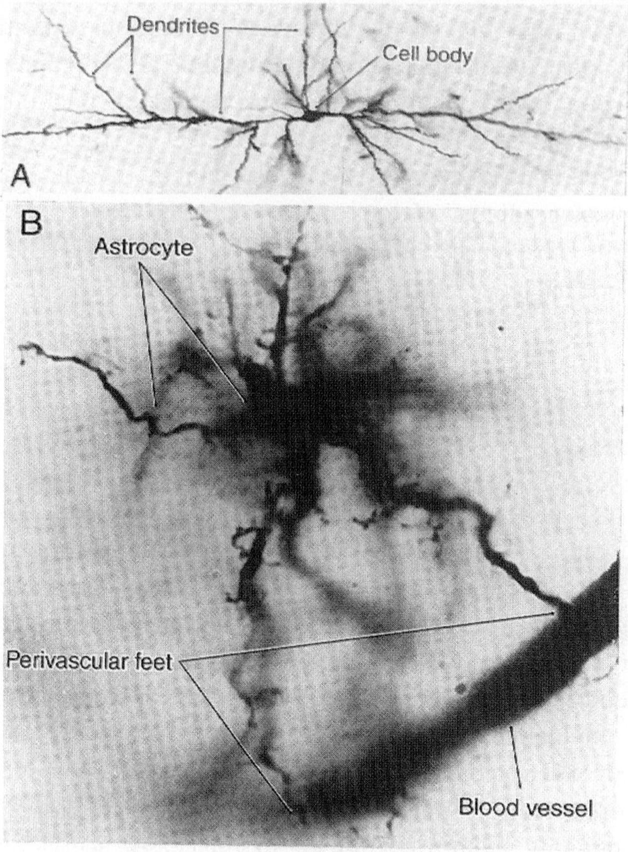

Figure 4. Neurons (A) and an astrocyte (B) in the central nervous system. (Reprinted from[1])

microglia. Each of them performs unique functions. Oligodendrocytes form myelin sheaths to insulate the nerve fiber so that they assure the speed of an action potential. The thickness of the myelin sheath has been linked to the speed of conduction.[7] In the peripheral nervous system, nerve fibers are encapsulated by Schwann cells. Astrocytes are star-like cells. It has been shown that processes in astrocytes are in extensive contact with neurons and blood vessels. As indicated by this convenience, astrocytes are actively involved in neurotransmitter metabolism, ionic regulation, scar formation and the BBB regulation. Microglia that are quiescent under normal condition, however, become active upon inflammation/injury. Similar to macrophages, active microglia migrate to the injury site, proliferate, and phagocytose microbes/damaged cells and tissues.

2. Epidemiology, Etiology and Pathophysiologies of Neurological Disorders

As complicated as its structure, the nervous system suffers from a variety of neurological disorders. The scope of this chapter will cover three categories which include neurotrauma, neurodegenerative diseases and autoimmune diseases are represented by one disorder in each category.

2.1. Spinal Cord Injury

Spinal cord injury is a major type of neurotrauma that mainly targets the young population between 16 and 30. According to the national spinal cord injury database, 23,683 persons suffered from it by June, 2005.[8] People who survived the trauma have to cope with life-long disabilities ranging from paraplegia to quadriplegia depending on the location of the injuries. The higher the location, the more a region will be affected so cervical injury will result in quadriplegia. In clinical conditions, the spinal cord is seldom severed physically, however, the cord below the injury losses the functions partially or completely.

Usually, the spinal cord injury is initiated by mechanical forces that dislocate the vertebral column. The fractured bone compresses rather than severs the cord. As the cord is compressed cross-sectionally, the gray matter and white matter deform and are pushed both upwards and downwards (Fig. 5). Moreover, the center of the cord deforms worse compared to the outside leaving only the border of cord intact.[9] During the surgery, dislocated bone chips are removed and sometimes, the compressed cord regains its normal shape but not its function. The deformation of the cord together with the disruption of vascular structures around the cord triggers secondary injury mechanisms which could last from several weeks to months. This chronic stage of SCI has been viewed as a neurodegenerative disease as they share many processes.[10] Several important aspects of these secondary injury processes will be discussed here.

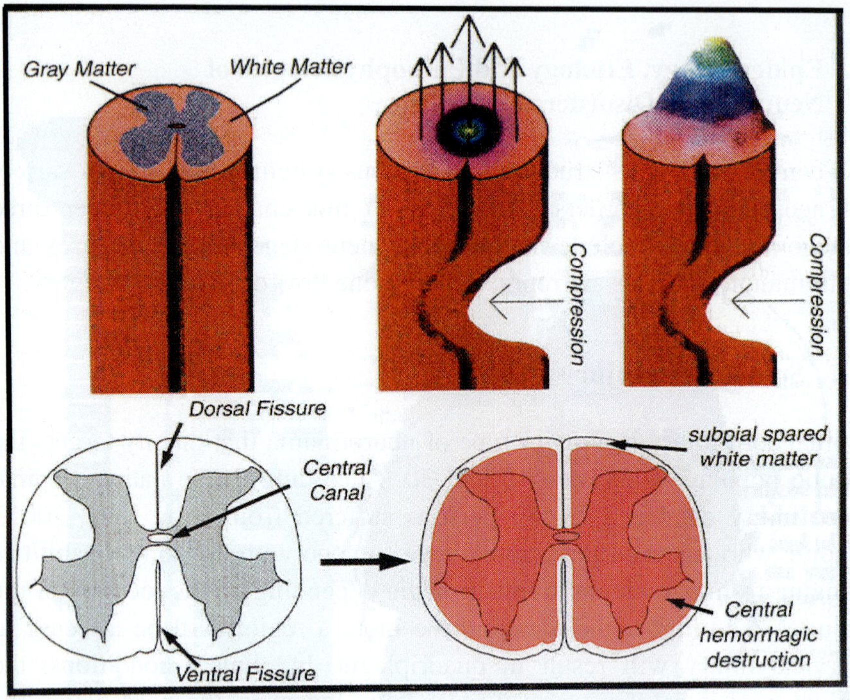

Figure 5. Pathology of SCI. (Reprint from[9])

Due to mechanical intrusion to the cord, the membranes of cells and their axons become permeable to various sizes of molecules.[11] Ions across membranes are tightly regulated under normal conditions. However, upon spinal cord injury, they move down their chemical gradient because of increased permeability. Ionic imbalance (especially K^+ and Na^+) depolarizes the neuron membrane so that the neuron is not capable of generating and conducting an action potential.[12] Thus, the information flow in both directions is disrupted. Over time, the axons go through demyelination and Wallerian degeneration and, in the end, axotomy. The nervous system is separated into two parts by the injury so the patient loses sensations as well as voluntary and involuntary control of muscles. One important message from the spinal cord injury is that paralysis is largely due to the loss of this axonal connection rather than neuron death.[9]

Ionic disturbances can also be induced by excitotoxicity.[13] Glutamate, the most abundant excitatory amino acid in the CNS, is stored in the vesicles near the presynaptic terminal ending. It releases into the synaptic cleft when the membrane is depolarized. The receptors to glutamates include both metabotropic and ionotropic ones. They work together leading to massive invasion of Ca^{2+}, K^+ and Na^+ when glutamate accumulates in the cleft.

Ionic imbalance also impairs the mitochondria functions causing overproduction of free radicals.[14,15] Free radicals are very unstable. Usually, they convert into another free radical species or more stable molecules such as lipid peroxidation (LPO) products which contribute to carbonyl stress.[16] Since the lipid peroxidation reaction is self-propagating, the concentration of LPO products increases following injury. These carbonyl products react with DNAs, proteins and carbohydrates leading to abnormal functioning of these macromolecules. If the injury progresses without interruption, neurons in the nervous system will die through either apoptosis or necrosis. Differences between these two have been reviewed at [17].

2.2. Alzheimer's Disease

Alzheimer's disease (AD) is an age-related neurodegenerative disease. It has been the most common condition that accounts for senile dementia. Its occurrence increases with age, however, it could happen in those below sixty five years old. Some cases especially in the early onset form have shown genetic involvement such as autosomal dominant disease, but a majority of these cases are sporadic. Thus, Alzheimer's disease is a heterogeneous disease that both genetic and environmental factors are possibly involved.[18]

Its diagnosis is based on both clinical and pathological evidence. The patients display impaired short and long term memory and abstract thinking. The symptoms continue aggravating over time from mild, medium to severe. As the disease progresses, patients could possibly display significant changes in their personality. Clinical diagnoses have to rule out other possibilities; however, the result is not always clean cut. The only definitive diagnosis is post-mortem histological exam of brain tissue. Two neuropathological characteristics for Alzheimer's diseases are senile plaques and neurofibrillary tangles (Fig. 6). The senile plaques also called amyloid plaques consist of a core of β-amyloid proteins which are insoluble therefore accumulate in the brain. Unlike β-amyloid plaques unique to Alzheimer's disease, the neurofibrillary tangles have been observed in several other pathological conditions involving dementia.[18] They are composed of microtubule associated proteins (tau) twisted into a paired helical structure. Different from normal tau proteins, the tau proteins in the tangle are highly phosphorylated and accumulate inside the neurons. Several other neurochemical markers such as acetylcholine, norepinephrine, and somatostatin decrease in the patients, however, these might be subsequent to the neuron loss in the cerebral cortex and hippocampus.

The mechanism that causes Alzheimer's disease is still not clear. Several theories have been hypothesized. The gene accounting for familial Alzheimer's disease has been identified at chromosome 21.[19] However, this is not the same gene encoding β-amyloid protein (β-AP). β-amyloid protein is an alternative splicing product from β-amyloid precursor protein (β-APP) which expresses extensively in a variety of tissues including neural tissue and codes for several amino acids. One of them with 695 amino acids is dominant in brain. It is still a myth what triggers the abnormal metabolism of β-APP. It is also interesting to find out that the protein aggregation/deposition is a wide spread phenomenon among various neurological disorders such as β-AP and phosphorylated tau in AD, α-synuclein in Parkinson's disease and huntington in Huntington's disease.[20-22] Recent research has indicated that the risk factors for cardiovascular diseases such as diabetes, high cholesterol,

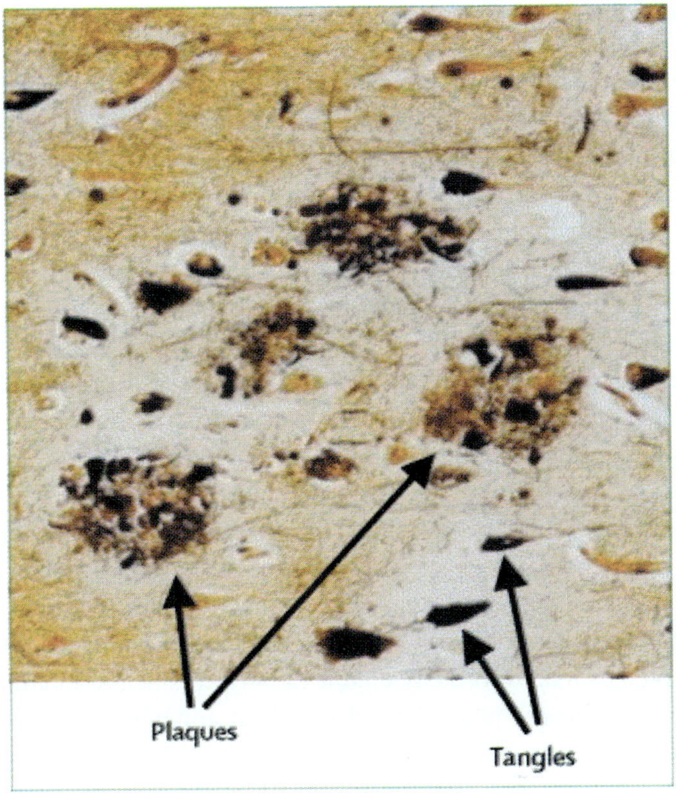

Figure 6. Beta-amyloid protein plaques and tau neurofibrillary tangles in the cerebral cortex of a patient with Alzheimer's disease (reprinted from[19]).

high blood pressure increases the odds for AD.[23] This may indicated that proteins aggregation is the result of abnormal metabolism, gene susceptibilities and environmental factors. It should be noted that β-AP and tau neurofibrillary tangle are both toxic to neurons. So once the trigger is pulled, these processes keep rolling and engage in self-propagation. β-amyloid protein in the meantime can be detected in the normal brain but at a lower level which suggests that the onset of AD might be the continuing changes like normal aging but with acceleration once overcoming a critical level.

2.3. Multiple Sclerosis

Multiple sclerosis (MS) is a neurological disorder targeting especially the white matter in the central nervous system (such as optic nerve, spinal cord and cerebrum). Therefore, peripheral nerves have been spared from this disease. MS differs a lot among patients in both its clinical symptoms and its progression, which makes it really difficult to diagnose each case with certainty.[24] Usually, patients experience their first symptoms in their 20s to 40s. At its early acute stage, MS exhibits an unpredictable pattern of occurring and disappearing, which is the so called relapsing-remitting (RR) MS. As the disease progresses to the chronic stage, more than half of patients suffer more severe physical disabilities, depression and mild cognitive impairment.

Under a microscope, the MS affected tissues from RR patients display a vague boundary of lesions, invasive infiltration of lymphocytes through parenchyma, loss of oligodendrocytes. Myelin (Fig. 7A), the primary target of the acute stage, has changed from its normal lamellar shape into vesicular structures.[25] But the most important is the abundance of macrophages that vigorously engulf the myelin sheath. In contrast, the lesions in the chronic phase have formed an apparent edge with naked axons embedded in scar tissue formed by astrocytes. Myelin has dissolved into droplets and has been phagocytosed by macrophages (Figure 7B).

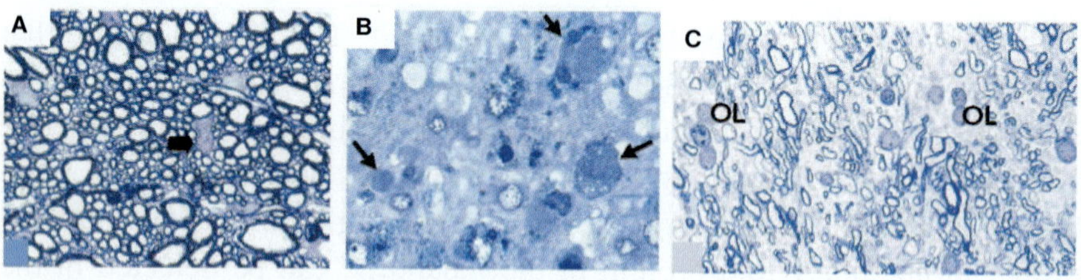

Figure 7. Multiple sclerosis in human tissue. A. Normal tissue. B. The active lesions of multiple sclerosis. C. The chronic lesion of multiple sclerosis (reprint from[25]).

The differences between the acute and chronic stages of MS raise the possibility that different mechanisms are responsible for each stage.[26] In the acute stage, unknown factors activate myelin-reactive T cells with TH1-mediated response. B cells undergo proliferation and somatic mutation, a process known for antigen recognition. Thus, patients experience systemic immune responses. However, in the chronic progressive stage, the inflammatory response is more localized which could explain why the temporal evolution of MS is heterogeneous and the inefficacy of immunoregulatory therapies in the chronic stages. Recently, it has been proposed that apoptotic death of oligodendrocytes causes molecular changes in the myelin sheath followed by recruitment of systemic immune responses targeting the myelin sheath.

But the factor(s) that initiate MS is still unknown. Epidemiological studies have shown MS has a pattern of family aggregation.[24] Monozygotic twin has 25 to 30% chance of developing MS when one of them is diagnosed compared to 191 in 100,000 in the white US population. In addition, they tend to display similar symptoms when MS is generally phenotypically heterogeneous. Besides the genetic factor, it has also been found that people who live further away from the equator are generally more susceptible to MS and women are more susceptible than men by 2:1. But MS in men tend to be more severe and aggressive than in women. So the results indicated that multiple factors rather than a single one contribute to the pathogenesis of MS.

3. Current Clinical Therapies and Limitations

All of these neurological disorders have great social-economic impacts. Central nervous system (CNS) trauma and MS happen to people early in their lives and usually leave them with various degree of disability. Not only do they have to learn from the beginning how to cope with the challenges in their daily lives but they also need great emotional and physical support from their families and communities. SCI and its related conditions cost the nation around $10 billion each year. Even though the affected population is smaller than the neurodegenerative diseases, the average lifetime cost for an individual with SCI is estimated to be at least $600,000, three times of that for AD due to increasing life expectancies.[5] On the other hand, neurodegenerative diseases such as Alzheimer's disease usually hit people in their 60's. As the disease progresses, patients need family care and even professional care. It has been estimated that the direct and indirect costs of AD nationwide are $100 billion annually.[27] The average age of America is rising continuously. More than half of the population will be older than 45 by 2010.[28] As the baby boomer generation is moving to their 50's and 60's, the cases for neurodegenerative diseases are expected to reach all time highs.

The calls for clinical treatments for CNS trauma and neurodegenerative disorders keep rising because of the increased public awareness as well as private and governmental support groups. The goal is to improve the quality of life for patients and alleviate the emotional and financial stresses on their families and society. Without expanding the knowledge of pathogenesis of these disorders over last few decades, clinical research could not have made it this far but there is still a long way ahead to research such diseases in order to cure them.

3.1. Approved Treatments of SCI and Ongoing Human Clinical Trials

Clinical research on spinal cord injury has been quite active since the 1980's. But there is only one FDA approved pharmacological treatment with methylprednisolone given within the first 8 hours after injury.[29] Many treatments have moved from clinical animal models to human clinical trials in the last few years. A discussion on clinical trials focusing on reducing spinal cord injury complications is beyond the scope of this book. Three major therapeutic strategies to improve a patient's sensory and motor function recoveries will be reviewed here.

The first (also most popular) one is to stimulate nerve regeneration by various means such as electrical fields. A joined research team from Purdue University and Indiana University has finished phase I human clinical trials to test a device called an oscillating field stimulator (OFS). In a paper published in January, 2005 in the *Journal of Neurosurgery Spine.*, the researchers claimed that OFS is safe and reliable.[30] Compared to a National Acute Spinal Cord Injury Studies (NASCIS) III study, they also shown efficacy. Currently they are trying to evaluate motor functional recovery by recruiting more patients.

The second approach is to implant a neuroprosthesis to improve a patient's specific muscular functions. There are two independent human clinical trials currently conducted by Toronto Rehabilitation Institute and Case Western Reserve University. Given the acknowledge that the device still needs to be improved, the concept of neuroprosthesis together with other traditional treatments is very promising for spinal cord injury rehabilitation.

The last but also the most challenging and controversial method is to use appropriate interventions to regulate secondary injury processes as they are responsible for the exasperation of injury. Manipulating natural body responses to the initial injury turns out to be very tricky. Many ion channel blockers and glutamate receptor antagonists have failed in human clinical trials because they either failed to show efficacy or triggered undesirable side effects.[31] Recently, Procord started recruiting patients for their phase II human clinical trials using autologous incubated macrophages. Even though it raised a lot of controversial comments from peers, their phase I trial reported preliminary efficacy of improving functional recovery and no side effects relevant to the procedure.[32] It would be desirable to review their results from phase II human clinical trials as this represents a unique approach to treat spinal cord injury and opens the door to its application on other neurological disorders such as multiple sclerosis.

3.2. Pharmacological Treatments of Alzheimer's Disease and Ongoing Human Clinical Trials

Treatment of AD is broadly divided into two classes. One targets the symptoms and the other the mechanisms, although some of the treatments to be discussed here aim at both. Most current treatments available to patients with Alzheimer's disease target its symptoms not mechanisms. Thus, they can not stop or slow down the progression of AD. Among those are cholinesterase inhibitors, N-methyl-d-aspartate antagonists, neurotrophic factors, and hormone replacement therapy.

Donepezil is a cholinesterase inhibitor (ChEI) which has been shown to slow down the decline in cognition, functional activities and behavior.[33] With potential long-term medication given to patients, it imposes safety concerns as well.

As the pathology of AD resembles chronic inflammation and the application of anti-inflammatory agents reduce the β-AP in the brain by inhibiting β- and γ-secretase activities to improve cognitive function in the animal models, several non-steroid anti-inflammation drugs (NSAIDs) such as indomethacin and diclofenac have moved to human clinical trials. Although small pilot studies reported positive results, much longer and larger trials using other NSAIDs (i.e., naproxen, rofecoxib) did not pass efficacy tests.[34,35]

Mechanism-oriented treatments are pursued based on the belief that β-AP metabolism is disrupted, which causes accumulation and agglomeration of excessive amounts of β-AP outside of neurons in the brain. It has been proposed that two mechanisms could account for this. Either the immune system could not effective deal with it or the production of β-AP is out of control. Immunotherapy (active and passive) is to boost the immune response to take up β-AP more efficiently and remove it from the brain or prevent β-AP from polymerization and, thus, precipitating in the tissue. Even though phase II clinical trials of AN-1792 (amyloid vaccine) failed because of the development of meningoencephalitis in 18 of 298 (6%) patients, this approach is still promising when proper caution is taken.[36]

It is well-known that insoluble β-AP derived from β-APP is closely related to the pathogenesis of AD. At least it has been carefully studied in autosomal dominant AD. This group of approaches includes the application of β-AP binding drugs such as Tramiprosate to prevent β-AP plaque formation to the reduction of β-AP synthesis by modulating key enzymes. Tramiprosate is currently under phase III trials as phase II trials have shown reduced β-AP plaque formation consistent with the improvement in cognition and global performance.[37] There are two key enzymes in the β secretase and the γ-secretase in the β-AP synthesis pathway. The mutation of γ-secretase (Presenilins gene) leads to increased γ-secretase activity, which causes some autosomal dominant AD. It provides the rationale for the treatment involving γ-secretase inhibitors. LY450139 developed by Eli Lilly is an example of γ-secretase inhibitor that just passed phase I clinical trials.[38]

3.3. Pharmacological Treatments of Multiple Sclerosis (MS) and Ongoing Human Clinical Trials

Due to its heterogeneity, advances in MS treatment have been slow until the last few years. Based on its clinical progression, MS has been divided into four groups as relapsing remitting, secondary progressive, primary progressive and primary relapsing.[39] Even though it is not clear whether the similar pathological processes are responsible for all the clinical subtypes, they have clearly responded differently to clinical therapies, which is discussed in the following.

It is widely accepted that the autoimmune system plays an important role in its pathological processes. So the primary therapeutic developments have been focused on immunomodulation. The current therapies approved by the Food and Drug Administration (FDA) include Interferon (IFN)-β1b, (IFN)-β1a, glatiramer acetate (GA) and mitoxanthrone for relapsing-remitting MS and cyclophosphamide and mitoxannthrone for secondary progressive MS.[40] No treatment has been established for primary progressive MS yet.

Interferon (IFN)-β1b and IFN-β1a have similar biological properties with slight differences in their structures. Their putative immunomodulatory effects have been achieved in several ways such as down-regulation of pro-inflammatory cytokines and up-regulation of anti-inflammatory cytokines, inhibition of T-cell infiltration across BBB. Their clinical efficacy has proved to reduce the relapse rate, relapse severity and the onset of clinically definite MS within the observed time window. However, prolonged exposure to IFN- β will induce some degree of adaptation among the patients by the generation of neutralizing antibodies (NAbs).

For the patients with secondary progressive MS, mitoxantrone is the only available treatment. Its immunosuppressive mechanism is due to the inhibition of DNA repair and synthesis in non-dividing and dividing cells. It has been clinically proven to reduce the incidence of new lesions, number of relapses over time and progression rates of neurological disability. However, even it is rare; mitoxantrone can induce leukemias and cardiotoxicity.

The search for immunomudulators and immunosuppressors has yielded many promising results. Some drugs are currently tested for human clinical trials. They represent many ways to tackle the inflammatory processes. For example, FTY720 is a synthetic drug acting on sphinogosine-1 receptor so that it can trap T-cells in the lymph glands and reduce the infiltration of T-cells across the BBB. Phase II clinical trials have shown reduction in lesions, neurological disability and number of relapses[41].

At the early stage, patients experience transient neurological disabilities which will completely or partially recover later. However as the disease progresses, these neurological disabilities become irreversible, which indicates permanent cell death, axonal loss and an inability to remyelination. While most of clinical research is dedicated to an immune response, we have to realize that neuroprotection needs to be considered at this irreversible stage to improve functional recovery. Currently most of the research in this direction is still limited to the research level. There have been a few potential therapeutic targets supported by pathological evidence. Excitotoxicity has been involved in neuronal death and axon degeneration in a variety of diseases so this similarity could facilitate drug selection. Among them, voltage-dependent sodium channel and L-type calcium channel blockers have show protective effects on axon. On the other side, the nervous system, especially CNS, present a very pessimistic environment for axon regeneration. Thus, neurotrophic factors and the antibodies against myelin inhibitors (i.e. Nogo-A protein) are perfect candidates to help axonal regeneration. One of the major characteristic in MS is the demyelination of axons blocking action potentials and leaving them to the extracellular environment without protection. So remyelination is another key aspect of neuroprotection. Though transplantation of autologous Schwann cells has failed to achieve this, the implantation of synergenic adult neural stem cells have provided positive evidence for remyelination and functional improvement.[42,43]

Multiple sclerosis is a heterogeneous diseases reflected by its etiology, pathological progression, clinical response. Thus, it provides a basis for combination of different therapeutic strategies mentioned above.

4. Application of Nanotechnology on the Development of Novel Drug and Cell Delivery Systems for the Nervous System

4.1. Conventional Drug Delivery Systems and Their Limitations

Molecules such as drugs, peptides and genetically engineered materials have been introduced into the body by conventional delivery systems which consist of oral, intravenous, intraperitoneal, topical and inhaled formulations. However, conventional molecule delivery systems simply rely on the body to transport drugs so it is a passive system. This has been associated with many drawbacks. First of all, molecules are distributed in the body nonspecifically. Since many drugs have systemic effects other than local effects, unwanted side effects can haul their potential therapeutic applications in human clinics. For example, it is well known that glutamate-mediated excitoxicity is a key pathological process responsible for cell death in various neurological disorders and trauma. However, drugs such as NMDA antagonists that target glutamate-mediated excitotoxicity have not passed human clinical trials for stroke because they have no efficacy and have significant side effects.[44] The failure of this type of drug is due to an abundant distribution of glutamate receptors that respond to NMDA.

Second, drugs are subjected to hydrolysis, pH changes or enzymatic degradation continuously once they are introduced into the body. Therefore, they might not be able to reach an effective concentration or sustain an effective concentration long enough at an area of interest. One way to compensate for this is to increase drug dose which will increase side effects.

Third, the challenge of drug delivery to the CNS is tremendous. There are three levels of resistance from arachnoid tight junctions, choroid plexus and cerebral capillaries (BBB).[45] The BBB can block most drugs except small hydrophobic ones. One classic example is dopamine drug which was originally chosen to treat Parkinson's disease. But it can not pass through the BBB. L-Dopa therefore was substituted for dopamine since it can move across the BBB by an amino acid transporter, system L and be converted into dopamine in the brain.[46] But this conversion happens in the other tissues as well which leads to various side effects and reduces the amount of L-dopa available for the brain.[47] There are several other options to deliver molecules to the brain including changing the dose but all of them have drawbacks.

Lastly, the demand for gene and peptide therapy is increasing since they have shown promises in reversing several neurological disorders. Gene therapies have succeeded in treating several neurological disorders in animal models such as Parkinson's disease, Lysosome storage disorder, Alzheimer's disease (AD) and stroke and some have even been moved into human clinical trials.[48-50] But how to deliver genes to the brain can be challenging since the brain is protected by the skull and the BBB. Injecting virus vectors directly into an afflicted area by opening part of skull is a very invasive procedure that can not be conducted often because of the risk of the infection. However, intravenous delivery of virus vectors can not go through the BBB. Moreover, the design of virus vectors can be very tricky. If a vector has a limited infecting capability, it is unlikely to invade host cells. If a vector is very infectious, replication of the virus vector can trigger an immune response.[51]

4.2. Advances of Nanotechnology in Drug Delivery Systems

Lately, nanotechnology has been involved in the creation of smart nanomaterials and microdevices that can deliver molecules to the nervous system in an active way. Several novel delivery systems using nanotechnology and their applications are discussed here:

Superparamagnetic iron oxide nanoparticles (SPIONs) (Fig. 8) consist of an iron oxide core of 10 nm diameter coated either with organic or inorganic coatings to improve its biocompatibility and add functional groups.[52] SPIONs have been used for gene therapy, magnetic resonance imaging, hyperthermia and radiotherapy. An in vitro study has shown that SPIONs can pass through artificial and real BBB membranes by endocytosis.[53,54] The existence of SPIONs did not trigger any inflammatory responses in both in vitro and in vivo models.[55] Once an appropriate functional group is added to SPION, we can control the delivery of molecules by external electrical fields and functional group recognitions.

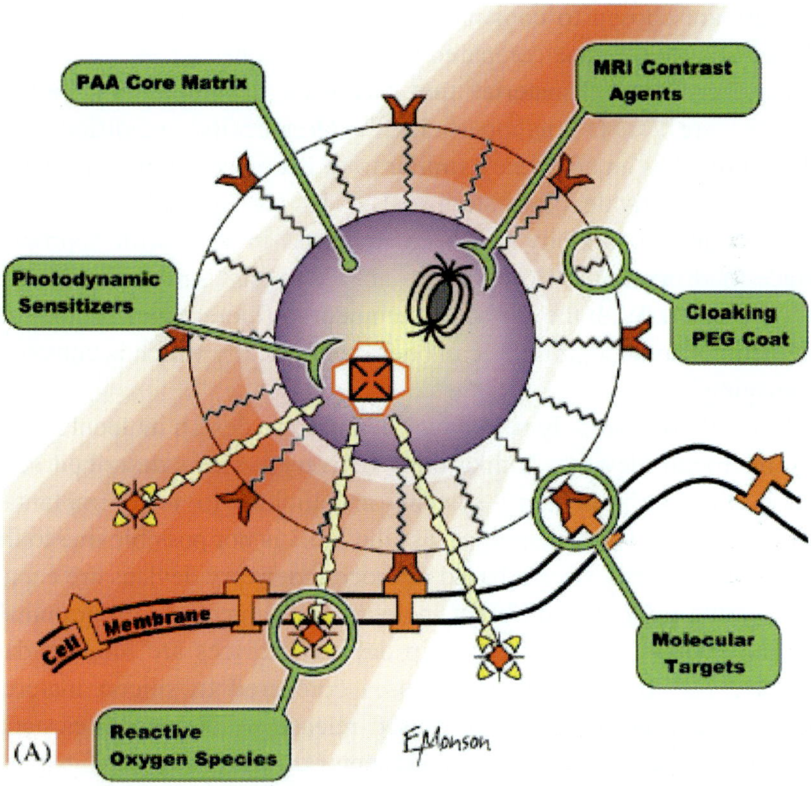

Figure 8. Multifunctional superparamagnetic iron oxide nanoparticles (SPIONs) (reprinted from[56]).

Polymer-based nanogels and nanoparticles have been used to deliver drugs, genes and antisenses and oligonucleotides.[57-59] Several studies have shown their ability to transport molecules across the BBB.[60,61] Depending on their preparation methods, the resulting polymers can be nanoparticles, nanospheres or nanocapsules. Several advantages are associated with polymer systems. Polymers are easy to synthesize and engineer with different functional groups to increase delivery specificity. Based on the polymer's properties (i.e. molecular weight and nature), we can control molecule release profiles.[62] Nanocapsules can also improve drug stability and bioavailability because they reduce unnecessary degradation of molecules at undesirable locations. When biodegradable polymers are chosen to construct a delivery system, it can sustain drug release for a longer time compared to the drug alone.[63]

Another type of material that has been developed for molecule delivery are silica nanoparticles.[64] Organically modified silica (ORMOSIL) has an efficiency similar to or even better than viral vectors for genes to activate brain stem cells.[65] Its biocompatibility has been improved and no toxicity has been observed in vivo with appropriate surface modification.[66] However, its ability to pass across the BBB has yet to be tested. With the surface attachment to fluorescence probes, cells that accumulate nanoparticles can be traced optically which is convenient for imaging.[67]

Both silicon and polymers have been used to design molecule release from microchip devices. Unlike other delivery systems described in this section, microchip delivery systems are limited to local implantable applications.[68,69] The transport across the BBB is not possible due to their microscale size. But silicon based microchip delivery devices are capable of delivering up to 100 different molecules in a precisely programmable fashion.[69] Polymer-based microchip delivery devices are biodegradable and have less inflammatory responses compared to silicon materials. They both can be designed for pulsed release which resembles natural hormone release patterns and avoid receptor down regulation.[70]

4.3. Nano-based Matrix for Stem Cell Delivery

Other than gene therapy, cell replacement therapy has promised a bright future to treat neurological disorders such as Alzheimer's disease and Parkinson's disease.[71, 72] There are three types of cell replacement therapies based on cell source. Cells can be either autologous or xenogeneic. Xenogeneic stem cells can be either adult stem cells or embryonic stem cells. Adult stem cells may not live long enough or proliferate as much as embryonic stem cells. Also adult stem cells have limited differentiating potentials compared to embryonic stem cells. The rarity of adult stem cells makes it difficult to access them. Adult stem cells do not behave in culture as predictably as do embryonic stem cells. They are more difficult to culture and maintain, and tend to spontaneously differentiate after a relatively short period of time. Because of these limitations, many scientists recommend embryonic stem cells. But the application of embryonic stem cells in cell therapy faces ethical challenges. For any cell source, an understanding of stem cell differentiation is a must for all applications. Factors that influence their differentiation include but are not restricted to physical, biochemical and genetic cues. With a good understanding of stem cell differentiation, we are able to control their differentiation in vitro and implant them into in vivo environments to replace damaged neural tissues.

Nano-based 3-D matrices made by different methods can mimic natural extracellular matrices so that we can study the proliferation and differentiation mechanisms of stem cells which will facilitate therapeutic applications. Two major classes of materials used to fabricate 3-D tissue scaffold are described here.

Polymers such as poly(L-lactic acid) (PLLA), collagen, gelatin and polycaprolactone (PCL) have been used to fabricate nano-structured porous tissue scaffolds by liquid-liquid phase separation and electrospinning methods.[73,74] In vitro studies have shown these 3-D porous scaffolds (Fig. 9) possess good biocompatibility.[74-76] Cell adhesion to materials can be enhanced further by surface functionalization of different molecules.[77,78] The characteristics of these scaffolds can be easily adjusted by changing fabrication parameters in order to meet different requirements. Besides polymers, self-assembling peptides have emerged as a promising new material. These nanostructures can create bulk materials with a variety of structural and functional properties dictated by their building blocks.[79] Unlike the solid tissue scaffolds made by other materials, peptides can assemble as an amorphous gel.[80] The transfer of stem cells can be achieved by a simple injection. Neural progenitor cells encapsulated by self-assembled tissue scaffolds have been shown to differentiate preferably into neurons rather than astrocytes. This indicates that the ability of self-assembled scaffolds to regulate cell differentiation by functionalizing them with different epitopes. Not only can peptide scaffolds regulate neural progenitor cell differentiation but they can also promote neurite regeneration.[81]

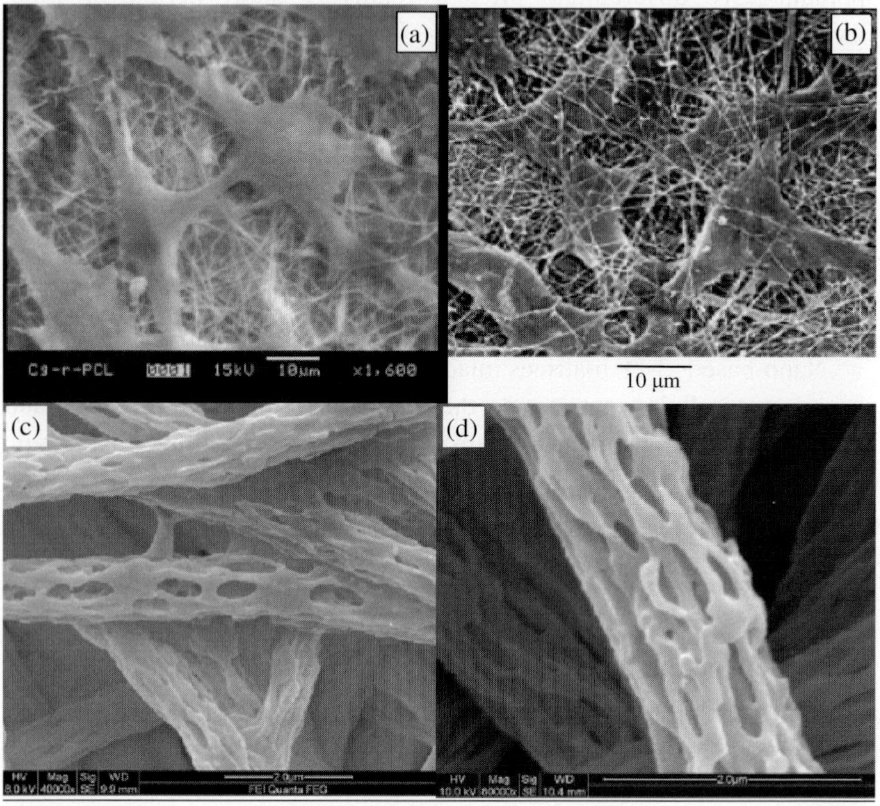

Figure 9. 3D nanofibers matrix for tissue engineering (reprinted from[75]).

4.4. Medical Imaging with Nanotechnology for Early Detection and Evaluation of Treatment

Medical imaging is a very powerful tool to help physicians diagnose diseases and formulate a better decision on disease treatment. Early detection of diseases will provide a window to slow down or stop diseases before they move into an irreversible stage.

Many nanosized medical imaging agents have a better signal to background ratio by functionalizing them with targeting molecules. With these target molecules, imaging agents mainly reach their target side by molecular recognition. These images have a better sensitivity and higher resolution.

Superparamagnetic iron oxide nanoparticles (SPIONs) have been mentioned in a previous section as a molecule delivery system. It is also a good MRI contrast enhancer. It detects tumors with higher sensitivity compared to conventional gadolinium administration (Fig. 10). Therefore, SPIONs can identify tumors that conventional imaging techniques could have missed.[82] Because of their nanosize, these SPIONs are able to pass through the BBB to identify brain tumors.[56,82] If the surgery navigation techniques can be combined with SPIONs, images of SPIONs can help neurosurgeons remove the tumor completely. As the polymer coatings on SPIONs can be conjugated to targeting moieties and fluorescence probes, SPIONs has the power to enhance imaging specificity and combine magnetic resonance imaging and fluorescence imaging.[83] SPIONs can not only improve brain tumor images but also kill tumor cells by hyperthermia.[84] When exposed to an alternating magnetic field, SPION induces heat. With target recognition, heat induction can be limited to the tumor tissue only.

Quantum dots are another promising material that can be used for diagnosis and imaging of brain tumors and neurological disorders. Their cores are nanometer sized semiconductor nanocrystals with polymer shells which can be conjugated to a variety of targeting molecules. The emission wavelength depends on the nature and size of quantum cores. Compared to conventional fluorescing molecules, quantum dots possess several attractive features. First, they have broad excitation spectra but very narrow emission spectra. For example, quantum dots with a CdSe-ZnS core-shell can be excited by the majority of the visible spectrum but emit within a narrow spectrum (FWHM ~ 30 to 45 nm).[85,86] Thus, it allows detection of various sizes of quantum dots with one wavelength. Second, quantum dots are resistant to photobleaching and exhibit bright

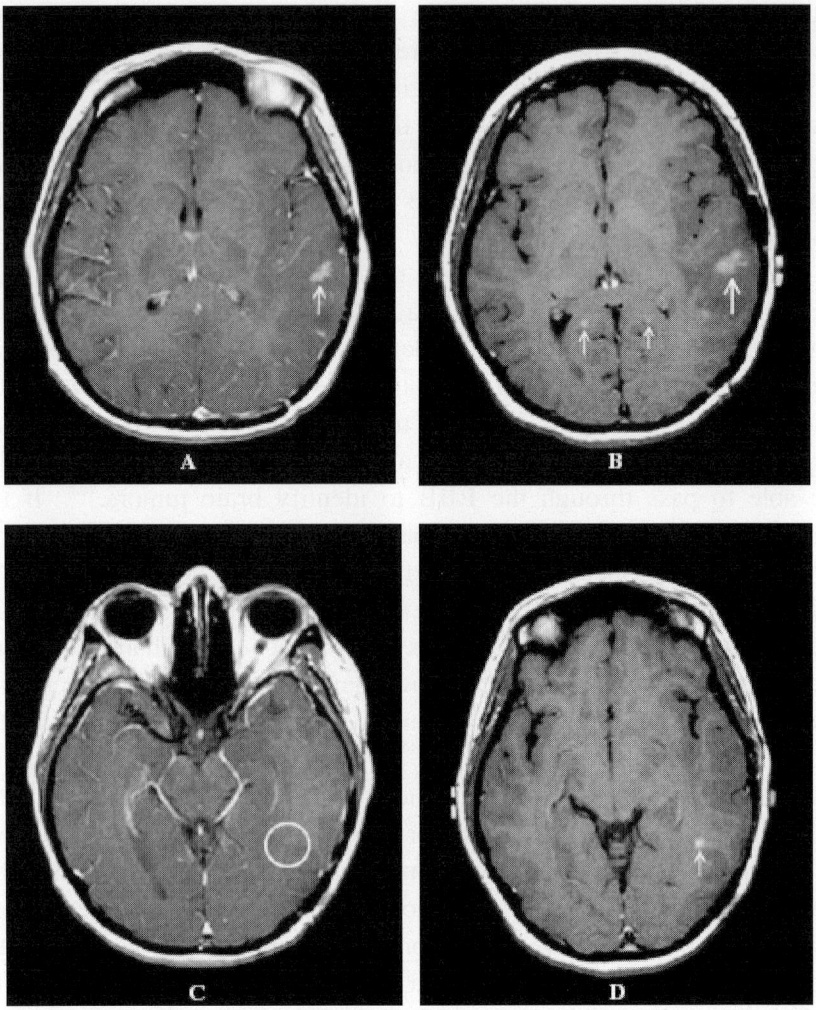

Figure 10. Imaging anaplastic oligodendroglioma (reprinted from[82]).

fluorescence.[87] Quantum dots can be applied not only to basic research to unveil secrets in CNS but also to clinical research such as neurological disorders and brain tumor diagnosis as well as their treatment evaluation. In addition, quantum dots can be potentially used for the design of visual prosthesis. In theory, quantum dot excitation can open ion channels and elicit action potentials in neurons when clusters of quantum dots get close to ion channels located on the cell membrane and create sufficient strengths of dipole moments.[88] Thus, the optical information can be converted into electrical signal and transmitted to the visual cortex.

By now, many delivery systems made of different nanomaterials have been introduced in this chapter. The advantages of these novel delivery systems synthesized by nanotechnology can be summarized as:

1. The size of delivery systems is at the same scale as that of cellular structures such as transporters, enzymes and cytoskeleton structures, which will facilitate the interactions between the synthetic systems with the cells.
2. Nanotechnology is able to modify the properties of individual building blocks to improve the performance of a delivery system. Coating the individual nanoparticles with polymers can not only reduce the toxicity of the delivery system but also extend its half-life in the circulation system.
3. The passage of therapeutic molecules through the BBB is not invincible any more. Their transport can be accomplished by receptor-mediated endocytosis of the delivery system without breaking down the BBB when the building block is conjugated to a molecule recognized by receptors located at the BBB.
4. By adding targeting molecules to the surface of a delivery system, we are able to deliver the therapeutic molecules to specific locations, therefore, this tailored delivery will improve the efficacy of therapeutic molecules and lower their systemic side effects.
5. The surface modifications of these delivery systems lead to the formation of multifunctional systems that can deliver therapeutic molecules, monitor and evaluate treatment efficacy.

5. Applications of Nanotechnologies in Electronic Tissue Interface Devices

As we have discussed in previous sections, many pharmacological approaches have either been tested or are being tested to stop or slow down the progression of various pathological processes of many neurological disorders successfully. Meanwhile, neuroprostheses which represent another broad range of electronic devices have appeared to be complementary approaches to regain to some extent lost functions due to illness and, thus, improve the quality of lives of patients whose conditions have progressed into irreversible stages (such as chronic cases of spinal cord injury), those who have no effective treatment available, and those who fail to respond to pharmacological treatments (such as for certain types of multiple sclerosis). Even though many neuroprostheses are still at their infancy, their preliminary success has presented an optimistic future.

The nervous system is an indispensable player for a human being to act as a synchronized unit and interact constantly with external and internal environments. The way our nervous system responds to external and internal stimuli can be comparable to a highway system with two-way traffic but our nervous system handles more traffic than any highway on the earth. The changes in the external environment picked up by sensory receptors are sent to the ascending pathway in the spinal cord via afferent peripheral nerves. The highway system of the spinal cord transports this important information up to different levels of the brain where information is analyzed and converted into command signals which are sent down via descending pathways into the spinal cord to motor neurons which leave the central nervous system and innervate different muscles. Thus, nerve impulses are changed into muscle contractions at neuron muscular junctions.

Neurological disorders can interrupt this information flow at various locations, therefore, neuroscientists have worked together with engineers to design various electronic devices that are located intimately with human tissues to create new pathways in order to navigate blocked traffic. Therefore we define these types of devices as electronic tissue interface devices. However, numerous terminologies have been used for specific applications. Several electronic tissue interface devices will be discussed in this section.

5.1. Cochlear Implant (Bionic Ear)

The ear is a sensory organ to perceive acoustic information in the environment. The outer and middle ear collects and amplifies sound but it is not until the inner ear that sound waves are transformed into nerve pulses by mechanoreceptors, specifically the hair cells. The nerve pulses are conducted from the brainstem via the eighth cranial nerve to the temporal lobe of cerebral cortex. If the inner ear fails to convert sound waves into nerve pulses due to damage patients usually suffer from severe hearing loss to deafness.

Unlike a hearing aid which only amplifies the sound, a cochlear implant consists of five major components which are dedicated to mimicking critical steps in the natural hearing process.[89] Three external parts which include a microphone, a speech processor and a transmitter are able to pick up, arrange and transmit processed sound over a radio frequency which is received by a receiver/transducer located underneath the skin. Sound information is converted into electrical signals by the receiver /transducer and is conducted by an electrode array which is inserted into the cochlear during surgery. There are more than 10,000 hair cells in the inner ear, but a modern cochlear implant contains a few more than 20 electrodes.[90] So, a lot of sound information is lost during speech processing. Patients need professional help to become accustomed to the sound created by a cochlear implant after surgery. Response to a cochlear implant varies from these who can communicate without a problem to those who need to employ lip-reading during conversation. So far this type of cochlear implant works better for speech than music.[91] Several other auditory prototype prostheses are available but need a few more years before their commercial versions reach clinical stage.[92,93]

5.2. Visual Prosthesis (Bionic Eye)

Signal transduction in the eye is similar to the ear in which image information is collected and focused by several optical components in an eye, converted into electrical signals by the retina and then transmitted to the visual cortex. Unlike the clinical success of cochlear implants, all of the visual prostheses are still under extensive preclinical research due to the complexity of visual perception. There are several designs of visual prostheses depending on their operating mechanisms. Similar to the assumption of a cochlear implant, the visual pathway beyond the retina including the optic nerve and the visual cortex is assumed to remain intact. A visual cortex prosthesis consists of a digital video camera system, a computer and an electrode array placed on the surface of visual cortex tissue.[94,95] A visual image captured by a digital video camera is decoded by a computer into a pattern of electrical stimulation which creates a sensation of a coarse pattern of light corresponding approximately to the topographical map of the visual cortex. In epiretinal prostheses, a photodiode chip is located behind the retina. A digital video camera captures an image which is processes by a computer and sent to an infrared LED screen. The light pattern on this LED screen is converted into a pattern of electronic signals by a photodiode chip.[96] Inner retinal cells which reside next to the photodiode chip pick up signals and transmit them to the visual cortex. Additionally, another type visual prosthesis has been developed by stimulating optic nerves.[97] Overall, current visual prostheses can help in short term blind patient to identify only lines, simple shapes and some characters. The true experience of sight is far from being realized.

5.3. Computer Brain Interface (BrainGate Technology)

Many neurological disorders can affect people's mobility such as multiple sclerosis (MS), amyotrophic lateral sclerosis (ALS), Parkinson's disease (PD) and spinal cord injury (SCI). Their difficulty in mobility can range from being incapable of gripping objects and speaking to not being able to move their arms and legs. Computer brain interface technology offers a great opportunity for these patients using their minds to escape their physical limitations. One type of technology called braingate takes advantage of the fact that patterns of intention-driven neural activities in the primary motor cortex still exist in patients who suffer from spinal cord injury.[98] A 96-microelectrode array (Fig. 11) is placed on the surface of the primary motor cortex and electrodes penetrate into the intermediate layers for recording purpose. After a patient imagines his limb motion such as moving a computer cursor through a mouse, cortical neuron spiking patterns are picked up by electrodes and are sent to a computer for decoding. A patient's motion intent is converted into control signals after neural signals are processed. Ideally, a patient can manage various tasks on a computer such as sending email and turning a television on without moving his/her body. Similar brain computer interfaces have been developed by other research groups and can help patients to accomplish similar tasks with or without visual and auditory cues.[99] A computer brain interface has also been tested to control prosthetic limbs.[100] Even though at the current stage of research the performance of the computer brain interface still needs to overcome many technical obstacles before patients can use it independently to communicate with the outside world, the concept of using the mind to communicate with the outside of world has proven feasible. The power of the computer brain interface devices is that when it combines with functional electrical stimulators (FES), patients can use their mind to regain control of many motor functions lost as a result of spinal cord injury and multiple sclerosis.[101]

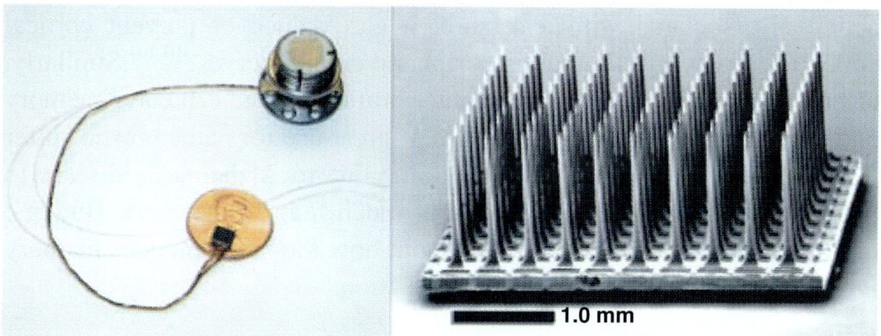

Figure 11. A BrainGate sensor and a SEM image of electrodes on the sensor (reprinted from[98]).

5.4. Functional Electrical Stimulation (FES)

Unlike the computer brain interface devices which use "mind" to control movements, FES devices restore motor functioning by directly stimulating the peripheral nerves. The nerve pulses are converted into muscle contraction at neuromuscular junctions. When the electrical signals is programmed in a certain way, muscle contractions can produce meaningful movements. Electrodes are placed on the skin or implanted in the muscle. Thus, the output electrical signals from the computer brain interface can control FES devices and consequently muscle contraction. This setup has been shown to restore hand grasp motion in a patient with tetraplegia.[102] More importantly, many muscles that are controlled by parasympathetic and sympathetic nerves can be controlled by mind too. Thus, patients can restore breathing function, bladder and bowel control, etc.[101]

5.5. Memory and Cognitive Functions

So far, all of the computer brain interface devices mentioned have been used to "read" the mind and transform such signals into a specific action. But in theory, we can also reverse the direction of signal transduction. This concept can be used to prevent certain types of seizures. Once the computer brain interface detects particular patterns of cortical neural activities associated with a seizure, it can reduce or prevent cortical epileptic activity by stimulating peripheral cranial nerves.[103,104] Similarly, electrical signals sent from a computer brain interface can carry memory and cognitive information. Thus, it is of great use for patients who suffer from memory loss and cognitive decline due to Alzheimer's disease to maintain day-to-day activities without much help from others. But first of all, we have to understand more about how the brain encodes memory information and maintains cognitive function.

5.6. Oscillating Field Stimulator (OFS)

OFS is one of few devices that actively interact with tissue among electronic devices used in the nervous system. OFS has three pairs of electrodes and are sutured to paravertebral musculature around spinal cord lesions. OFS provides an electrical field and alternate its polarity at a certain interval. Since neurons grow towards the cathode, injured neurons can regenerate towards both directions under the guidance of an oscillating electrical field. By encouraging injured neurons to grow across the lesion, OFS has been shown to improve sensory recovery in both human and animal studies.[105,106] But the window for OFS implantation is limited. Chronic spinal cord injuries does not respond as well as acute ones.[105]

6. How Can Nanotechnology Improve Performance of Electronic Tissue Interface Devices?

The proof of concept of electronic tissue interface devices presents an optimistic future to restore a disabled person's cognitive, communication and motor functions. But scientists and engineers need to work as a team to understand how the brain encodes and decodes a variety of information and tackle many technical obstacles before a working system like the cochlear implant is available to achieve its ultimate goal.

Most electronic tissue interface devices send and receive electrical signals from the nervous tissues via an array of electrodes which are usually composed of platinum, silicon or silicon rubber. Electrode array stability is a key to the long-term usage of these devices such as visual prostheses and computer-brain interfaces because of sophisticated and limited accesses to the nervous system. Repetitive surgery will increase the risk of infection and other complications. Currently, these devices except cochlear implants have only been tested for short-term applications.[98.106] Electrodes often fail to perform over time due to accumulation of astrocytes (so called gliosis) and neuron cell death around the electrodes or electrochemical reactions at the interface.[107,108] A reliable electrode recording requires not only the stability of electrode itself (reduction of electrochemical degradation and dielectric layers growth) but also favorable cell responses (stimulation of neurons and inhibition of glia).

Different nanotechnologies have been developed to solve these problems. For example, carbon nanotubes (CNT) may be an attractive material for electrodes because of their chemical stability, low resistance, and high charge capacitance.[109-111] Bonding of CNT to metals by ultrasonic nanowelding has been shown to decrease contact resistance, have good long-term stability and mechanical strength.[112] The availability of carbon nanotube chemical functionalization techniques allows CNT to detect not only electrical signals but also metabolic activity and enzymatic activity.[113]

Additionally, the biocompatibility of electrodes is very important to ensure stable recording in long-term implanted applications and physical bonding of electrodes to neuron tissue. Electrodes currently used for electronic tissue interface devices have a conventional (microscale) surface roughness which is not favorable for protein adsorption. In contrast, the extracellular matrix where neurons grow possesses nanoscale features due to, for example, proteins, lipids and carbohydrates. It has been shown that nano-surface roughness of silicon substrate (a typical material for electrodes) can increase the adhesion of neuron but decrease the adhesion of astrocytes (Fig. 12).[114] Chemical functionalization, neurotrophic factors and peptide coating of electrodes can also improve electrode biocompatibility by regulating both neuron and astrocyte adhesion on electrodes.[115-117]

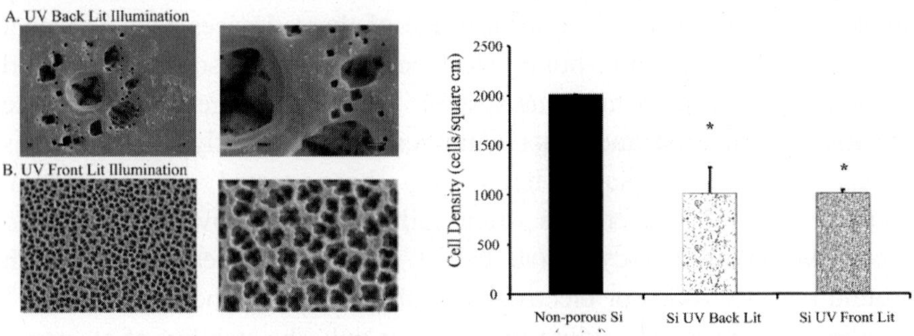

Figure 12. SEM images of nanoporous silicon created by (A) UV back lit and (B) UV front lit illumination and decreased astrocyte adhesion on nanoporous silicon (reprinted from[114]).

Signal transduction in the nervous system is accomplished by a large number of neurons and other types of cells such as sensory receptors. For example, there are 3,500 inner hair cells and 12,000 out hair cells in the ear and 1,200,000 axons in the optic nerves.[118-120] Although neuroscientists have long realized large neural ensembles in the nervous system, traditional technologies can only provide an array with less than

100 electrodes.[118,119] Thus, such neuroprosthese can not provide desirable spatial and temporal resolutions. Clinical trials have shown that patients implanted with such neuroprosthese have a very limited ability to respond to complicated signals such as music, visual objects, etc.. Nanotechnology has its advantage to allow engineers to design a miniature array with thousands of submicro-sized electrodes.[120] Both electron beam and nanoimprint lithography can create electrode sizes ranging from 110 nm to 550 nm on a 0.25 mm^2 Si3N4-coated Si (100) substrate (Fig. 13).[121] With submicro-sized electrodes, we can ensure a redundant and overlapping recording or stimulation of a much larger population of neurons with much greater sensitivity. It will also help to stabilize the placement of electrodes if low level electrical stimulation of neuron leads to the growth of neurites around the electrodes.[122]

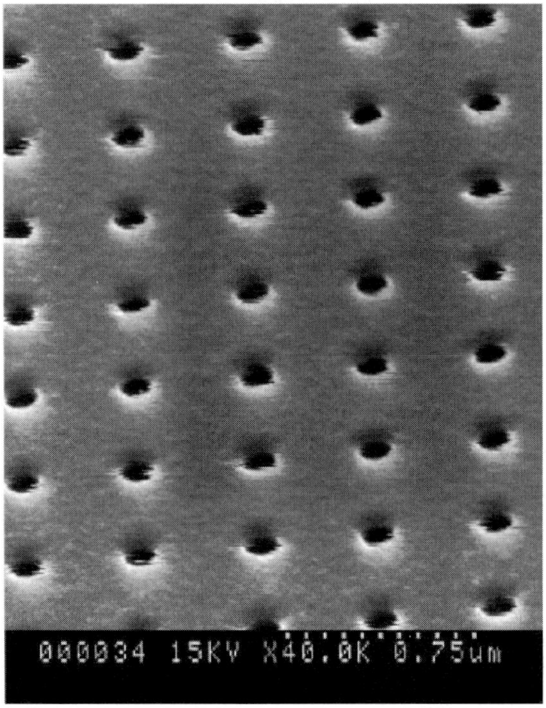

Figure 13. An example of nanoelectrode array produced by electron-beam lithography. (Reprint from[121])

Improving the performance, biocompatibility and stability of electrodes is just one aspect of what nanotechnology can contribute to the tissue electronic interface devices used in the nervous system. In addition, nanotechnology is capable of reducing the size of device and the signal acquisition and processing system. The miniature of devices makes a portable system possible for patients. Another critical factor to the mobility of the devices is the design of the battery and power source. Nanotechnology has been utilized to improve recharging time, longevity, size and weight of the power sources.[124,125] Discussion on the miniature device and battery, however, is beyond the scope of this chapter.

7. Future Directions and Considerations

The nervous system is a very complicated system with great plasticity. With the help of nanotechnology, neuroscientists, clinician, chemists and engineers have worked together as a team to tackle the challenges of the sophisticated nervous system. Nanotechnology has the potentials to help the successful translations of lab bench discoveries into bedside treatments for neurological trauma and disorders in many ways:

1. Applications of nanotechnology in basic neuroscience help us understand the principles of how the brain works under normal condition and etiologies and pathological processes of different diseases. Based on this basic research, we are able to identify potential therapeutic targets and design neuroprostheses that can interact with our nervous system better.
2. Because of its high sensitivity, nanotechnology can achieve early detection and diagnosis of neurological disorders and help us to make the right decision on strategies of treatments and stop the progress of diseases before they reach an irreversible stage
3. Before a new treatment or device is available for human, it has to be tested on an appropriate animal model. Nanotechnology can be used to evaluate the treatment in the animal models.
4. Whether a treatment is approved by food and drug administration (FDA) or not is dependent on both of its safety and efficacy. Either

fails will halt any efforts on its development. Nanotechnology has demonstrated its capability to improve efficacy, stability and reduce the toxicity of the therapeutic molecules.

Bibliography

1. Haines DE. (2002) *Fundamental Neuroscience, 2nd Edition*, Churchill Livingstone, London, pp. 28-35.
2. Alcamo EI and Krumhardt B. (2002) *Anatomy and Physiology the Easy Way, 2nd Edition*, Barron's Educational Series, Washington, D.C., pp. 226.
3. Schulze C, Firth JA. (1992) Interendothelial junctions during blood-brain barrier development in the rat: morphological changes at the level of individual tight junctional contacts. *Brain Res Dev Brain Res* **69(1)**: 85-95.
4. Smith MW, Gumbleton M. (2006) Endocytosis at the blood-brain barrier: from basic understanding to drug delivery strategies. *J Drug Target* **14(4)**: 191-214.
5. http://www.synapticusa.com/images/pathway_illust.jpg
6. Levitan IB, Kaczmarek LK. (1991) *The Neuron -- Cell and Molecular Biology*. Oxford University Press, Oxford. pp. 22-30, pp. 33-50.
7. Waxman SG. (1980). Determinants of conduction velocity in myelinated nerve fibers. *Muscle Nerve* **3(2)**: 141-50.
8. http://www.spinalcord.uab.edu/show.asp?durki=21446
9. Borgens RB. (2003) Restoring function to the injured human spinal cord. *Adv Anat Embryol Cell Biol* **71**: 1-155.
10. Bittigau P, Ikonomidou C. (1997) Glutamate in neurologic diseases. *J Child Neurol* **12(8)**: 471-85.
11. Luo J, Borgens R, Shi R. (2002) Polyethylene glycol immediately repairs neuronal membranes and inhibits free radical production after acute spinal cord injury. *J Neurochem* **83(2)**: 471-80.
12. Jensen JM, Shi R. (2003) Effects of 4-aminopyridine on stretched mammalian spinal cord: the role of potassium channels in axonal conduction. *J Neurophysiol* **90(4)**: 2334-40.
13. Choi DW. (1992) Excitotoxic cell death. *J Neurobiol* **23(9)**: 1261-76.
14. Dugan LL, Choi DW. (1994) Excitotoxicity, free radicals, and cell membrane changes. *Ann Neurol* **35**: S17-21.
15. Azbill RD, Mu X, Bruce-Keller AJ, Mattson MP, Springer JE. (1997) Impaired mitochondrial function, oxidative stress and altered antioxidant enzyme activities following traumatic spinal cord injury. *Brain Res* **765(2)**: 283-90.
16. Miyata T, Kurokawa K, Van Ypersele De Strihou C. (2000) Advanced glycation and lipoxidation end products: role of reactive carbonyl compounds generated during carbohydrate and lipid metabolism. *J Am Soc Nephrol* **11(9)**: 1744-52.

17. Nicotera P, Leist M, Ferrando-May E. (1999) Apoptosis and necrosis: different execution of the same death. *Biochem Soc Symp* **66**: 69-73.
18. Strange PG. (1992) *Brain Biochemistry and Brain Disorders.* Oxford University Press, Oxford, NY. pp. 210-213.
19. Blennow K, de Leon MJ, Zetterberg H. (2006) Alzheimer's disease. *Lancet* **368(9533)**: 387-403.
20. Stefani M, Dobson CM. (2003) Protein aggregation and aggregate toxicity: new insights into protein folding, misfolding diseases and biological evolution. *J Mol Med* **81(11)**: 678-99.
21. Sherer TB, Betarbet R, Greenamyre JT. (2001) Pathogenesis of Parkinson's disease. *Curr Opin Investig Drugs* **2(5)**: 657-62.
22. Bates G. (2003) Huntington aggregation and toxicity in Huntington's disease. *Lancet* **361(9369)**: 1642-4.
23. Whitmer RA, Sidney S, Selby J, Johnston SC, Yaffe K. (2005) Midlife cardiovascular risk factors and risk of dementia in late life. *Neurology* **64(2)**: 277-81.
24. Warren S, Warren KG. (2001) *Multiple Sclerosis.* World Health Organization, Geneva, pp. 7-15.
25. Frohman EM, Racke MK, Raine CS. (2006) Multiple sclerosis--the plaque and its pathogenesis. *N Engl J Med* **354(9)**: 942-55.
26. Barnett MH, Sutton I. (2006) The pathology of multiple sclerosis: a paradigm shift. *Curr Opin Neurol* **19(3)** :242-7.
27. http://www.alz.org/AboutAD/Statistics.asp
28. Toossi M. (2000) A century of change: the US labor force, 1950-2050. *Monthly Labor Review*.
29. Delamarter RB, Coyle J. (1999) Acute management of spinal cord injury. *J Am Acad Orthop Surg* **7(3)**: 166-75.
30. Shapiro S, Borgens R, Pascuzzi R, Roos K, Groff M, Purvines S, Rodgers RB, Hagy S, Nelson P. (2005) Oscillating field stimulation for complete spinal cord injury in humans: a phase 1 trial. *J Neurosurg Spine* **2(1)**: 3-10.
31. Prass K, Dirnagl U. (1998) Glutamate antagonists in therapy of stroke. *Restor Neurol Neurosci* **13(1-2)**: 3-10.
32. Knoller N, Auerbach G, Fulga V, Zelig G, Attias J, Bakimer R, Marder JB, Yoles E, Belkin M, Schwartz M, Hadani M. (2005) Clinical experience using incubated autologous macrophages as a treatment for complete spinal cord injury: phase I study results. *J Neurosurg Spine* **3(3)**: 173-81.
33. Gauthier SG. (2005) Alzheimer's disease: the benefits of early treatment. *Eur J Neurol* **Suppl 3**: 11-6.
34. Aisen PS, Schafer KA, Grundman M, Pfeiffer E, Sano M, Davis KL, Farlow MR, Jin S, Thomas RG, Thal LJ. (2003) Alzheimer's Disease Cooperative Study. Effects of rofecoxib or naproxen vs placebo on Alzheimer disease progression: a randomized controlled trial. *JAMA* **289(21)**: 2819-26.

35. Reines SA, Block GA, Morris JC, Liu G, Nessly ML, Lines CR, Norman BA, Baranak CC. (2004) Rofecoxib Protocol 091 Study Group. Rofecoxib: no effect on Alzheimer's disease in a 1-year, randomized, blinded, controlled study. Neurology. **62(1)**: 66-71.
36. Orgogozo JM, Gilman S, Dartigues JF, Laurent B, Puel M, Kirby LC, Jouanny P, Dubois B, Eisner L, Flitman S, Michel BF, Boada M, Frank A, Hock C. (2003) Subacute meningoencephalitis in a subset of patients with AD after Abeta42 immunization. *Neurology* **61(1)**: 46-54.
37. http://www.seniorjournal.com/NEWS/Alzheimer's/5-07-05Alzhemed.htm
38. Siemers ER, Quinn JF, Kaye J, Farlow MR, Porsteinsson A, Tariot P, Zoulnouni P, Galvin JE, Holtzman DM, Knopman DS, Satterwhite J, Gonzales C, Dean RA, May PC. (2006) Effects of a gamma-secretase inhibitor in a randomized study of patients with Alzheimer disease. *Neurology* **66(4)**: 602-4.
39. Lublin FD, Reingold SC. (1996) Defining the clinical course of multiple sclerosis: results of an international survey. National Multiple Sclerosis Society (USA) Advisory Committee on Clinical Trials of New Agents in Multiple Sclerosis. *Neurology* **46(4)**: 907-11.
40. Rizvi SA, Agius MA. (2004) Current approved options for treating patients with multiple sclerosis. *Neurology* **63(12 Suppl 6)**: S8-14.
41. http://www.medicalnewstoday.com/medicalnews.php?newsid=41281
42. Stangel M. (2004) Remyelinating and neuroprotective treatments in multiple sclerosis. *Expert Opin Investig Drugs* **13(4)**: 331-47.
43. Pluchino S, Quattrini A, Brambilla E, Gritti A, Salani G, Dina G, Galli R, Del Carro U, Amadio S, Bergami A, Furlan R, Comi G, Vescovi AL, Martino G. (2003) Injection of adult neurospheres induces recovery in a chronic model of multiple sclerosis. *Nature* **422(6933)**: 688-94.
44. Bentley P, Sharma P. (2005) Pharmacological treatment of ischemic stroke. *Pharmacol Ther* **108(3)**: 334-52.
45. http://www.usask.ca/anatomy/teaching/anat234/Lect2%20-BBB.pdf#search=%22anatomy%20of%20blood%20brain%20barrier%22
46. Kageyama T, Nakamura M, Matsuo A, Yamasaki Y, Takakura Y, Hashida M, Kanai Y, Naito M, Tsuruo T, Minato N, Shimohama S. (2000) The 4F2hc/LAT1 complex transports L-DOPA across the blood-brain barrier. *Brain Res* **879(1-2)**: 115-21.
47. http://www.wemove.org/bradykinesia/bra_tre.html
48. Luo J, Kaplitt MG, Fitzsimons HL, Zuzga DS, Liu Y, Oshinsky ML, During MJ. (2002) Subthalamic GAD gene therapy in a Parkinson's disease rat model. *Science* **298(5592)**: 425-9.
49. Mandel RJ, Burger C. (2004) Clinical trials in neurological disorders using AAV vectors: promises and challenges. *Curr Opin Mol Ther* **6(5)**: 482-90.
50. http://www.drugresearcher.com/news/ng.asp?n=58631-gene-therapy-reverses

51. Bangari DS, Mittal SK. (2006) Current strategies and future directions for eluding adenoviral vector immunity. *Curr Gene Ther* **6(2)**: 215-26.
52. Neuberger T, Schöpf B, Hofmann H, Hofmann M, Rechenberg B. (2005) Superparamagnetic nanoparticles for biomedical applications: possibilities and limitations of a new drug delivery system. *J Materials Magnetism* **293**: 483-496.
53. Mondalek FG, Zhang YY, Kropp B, Kopke RD, Ge X, Jackson RL, Dormer KJ. (2006) The permeability of SPION over an artificial three-layer membrane is enhanced by external magnetic field. *J Nanobiotechnology* **4**: 4.
54. Peira E, Marzola P, Podio V, Aime S, Sbarbati A, Gasco MR. (2003) In vitro and in vivo study of solid lipid nanoparticles loaded with superparamagnetic iron oxide. *J Drug Target* **11(1)**: 19-24.
55. Cengelli F, Maysinger D, Tschudi-Monnet F, Montet X, Corot C, Petri-Fink A, Hofmann H, Juillerat-Jeanneret L. (2006) Interaction of functionalized superparamagnetic iron oxide nanoparticles with brain structures. *J Pharmacol Exp Ther* **318(1)**: 108-16.
56. Kopelman R, Koo YL, Philbert M, Moffat BA, Reddy GR, McConville P, Hall DE, Chenevert TL, Bhojani MS, Buck SM, Rehemtulla A and Ross BD. (2005) Multifunctional nanoparticle platforms for in vivo MRI enhancement and photodynamic therapy of a rat brain cancer. *J of Magnetism and Magnetic Materials* **293**, 404-410.
57. McAllister K, Sazani P, Adam M, Cho MJ, Rubinstein M, Samulski RJ, DeSimone JM. (2002) Polymeric nanogels produced via inverse microemulsion polymerization as potential gene and antisense delivery agents. *J Am Chem Soc.* **124(51)**: 15198-207.
58. Vinogradov SV, Batrakova EV, Kabanov AV. (2004) Nanogels for oligonucleotide delivery to the brain. *Bioconjug Chem* **15(1)**: 50-60.
59. Kommareddy S, Amiji M. (2005) Preparation and evaluation of thiol-modified gelatin nanoparticles for intracellular DNA delivery in response to glutathione. *Bioconjug Chem* **16(6)**: 1423-32.
60. Roney C, Kulkarni P, Arora V, Antich P, Bonte F, Wu A, Mallikarjuana NN, Manohar S, Liang HF, Kulkarni AR, Sung HW, Sairam M, Aminabhavi TM. (2005) Targeted nanoparticles for drug delivery through the blood-brain barrier for Alzheimer's disease. *J Control Release* **108(2-3)**: 193-214.
61. Kreuter J, Ramge P, Petrov V, Hamm S, Gelperina SE, Engelhardt B, Alyautdin R, von Briesen H, Begley DJ. (2003) Direct evidence that polysorbate-80-coated poly(butylcyanoacrylate) nanoparticles deliver drugs to the CNS via specific mechanisms requiring prior binding of drug to the nanoparticles. *Pharm Res* **20(3)**: 409-16.
62. Cruz L, Soares LU, Costa TD, Mezzalira G, da Silveira NP, Guterres SS, Pohlmann AR. (2006) Diffusion and mathematical modeling of release profiles from nanocarriers. *Int J Pharm* **313(1-2)**: 198-205.

63. Panyam J, Labhasetwar V. (2004) Sustained cytoplasmic delivery of drugs with intracellular receptors using biodegradable nanoparticles. *Mol Pharm* **1(1)**: 77-84.
64. Bakalova R, Zhelev Z, Aoki I, Ohba H, Imai Y, Kanno I. (2006) Silica-shelled single quantum dot micelles as imaging probes with dual or multimodality. *Anal Chem* 2006 **78(16)**: 5925-5932.
65. Bharali DJ, Klejbor I, Stachowiak EK, Dutta P, Roy I, Kaur N, Bergey EJ, Prasad PN, Stachowiak MK. (2005) Organically modified silica nanoparticles: a nonviral vector for in vivo gene delivery and expression in the brain. *Proc Natl Acad Sci U S A* **102(32)**: 11539-44.
66. Jovanovic AV, Flint JA, Varshney M, Morey TE, Dennis DM, Duran RS. (2006) Surface modification of silica core-shell nanocapsules: biomedical implications. *Biomacromolecules* **7(3)**: 945-9.
67. Roy I, Ohulchanskyy TY, Bharali DJ, Pudavar HE, Mistretta RA, Kaur N, Prasad PN. (2005) Optical tracking of organically modified silica nanoparticles as DNA carriers: a nonviral, nanomedicine approach for gene delivery. *Proc Natl Acad Sci U S A* **102(2)**: 279-84.
68. Grayson AC, Choi IS, Tyler BM, Wang PP, Brem H,Cimal MJ and Langer R. (2003) Multi-pulse drug delivery from a resorbable polymeric microchip device. *Nat Mat* **2**: 767-772.
69. Prescott JH, Lipka S, Baldwin S, Sheppard NF Jr, Maloney JM, Coppeta J, Yomtov B, Staples MA, Santini JT Jr. (2006) Chronic, programmed polypeptide delivery from an implanted, multireservoir microchip device. *Nat Biotechnol* **24(4)**: 437-8.
70. http://ocw.mit.edu/NR/rdonlyres/AC67B859-F74E-4A3A-A417-0DCE69216294/0/BE462lect06.pdf#search=%22Lecture%206%3A%20Programmed%2FPulsed%20Drug%20Delivery%20and%20Drug%20Delivery%20in%20Tissue%20Engineering%22
71. Snyder BJ, Olanow CW. (2005) Stem cell treatment for Parkinson's disease: an update for 2005. *Curr Opin Neurol* **18(4)**: 376-85.
72. Sugaya K, Brannen CL. (2001) Stem cell strategies for neuroreplacement therapy in Alzheimer's disease. *Med Hypotheses* **57(6)**: 697-700.
73. Murugan R, Ramakrishna S. (2006) Nano-featured scaffolds for tissue engineering: a review of spinning methodologies. *Tissue Eng* **12(3)**: 435-47.
74. Yang F, Murugan R, Wang S, Ramakrishna S. (2005) Electrospinning of nano/micro scale poly(L-lactic acid) aligned fibers and their potential in neural tissue engineering. *Biomaterials* **26(15)**: 2603-10.
75. Zhang YZ, Feng Y, Huang Z-M, Ramakrishna S and Lim CT. (2006) Fabrication of porous electrospun nanofibres. *Nanotech* **17**: 901-908.
76. Ma W, Fitzgerald W, Liu QY, O'Shaughnessy TJ, Maric D, Lin HJ, Alkon DL, Barker JL. (2004) CNS stem and progenitor cell differentiation into functional neuronal circuits in three-dimensional collagen gels. *Exp Neurol* **190(2)**: 276-88.

77. Park YJ, Kim KH, Lee JY, Ku Y, Lee SJ, Min BM, Chung CP. (2006) Immobilization of bone morphogenetic protein-2 on a nanofibrous chitosan membrane for enhanced guided bone regeneration. *Biotechnol Appl Biochem* **43(Pt 1)**: 17-24.
78. Casper CL, Yamaguchi N, Kiick KL, Rabolt JF. (2005) Functionalizing electrospun fibers with biologically relevant macromolecules. Biomacromolecules. **6(4)**: 1998-2007.
79. Rajagopal K, Schneider JP. (2004) Self-assembling peptides and proteins for nanotechnological applications. *Curr Opin Struct Biol*. **14(4)**: 480-6.
80. Silva GA, Czeisler C, Niece KL, Beniash E, Harrington DA, Kessler JA, Stupp SI. (2004) Selective differentiation of neural progenitor cells by high-epitope density nanofibers. *Science* **303(5662)**: 1352-5.
81. Ellis-Behnke RG, Liang YX, You SW, Tay DK, Zhang S, So KF, Schneider GE. (2006) Nano neuro knitting: peptide nanofiber scaffold for brain repair and axon regeneration with functional return of vision. *Proc Natl Acad Sci U S A* **103(13)**: 5054-9.
82. Neuwelt EA, Varallyay P, Bago AG, Muldoon LL, Nesbit G, Nixon R. (2004) Imaging of iron oxide nanoparticles by MR and light microscopy in patients with malignant brain tumours. *Neuropathol Appl Neurobiol* **30(5)**: 456-71.
83. Veiseh O, Sun C, Gunn J, Kohler N, Gabikian P, Lee D, Bhattarai N, Ellenbogen R, Sze R, Hallahan A, Olson J, Zhang M. (2005) Optical and MRI multifunctional nanoprobe for targeting gliomas. *Nano Lett* 5(6): 1003-8.
84. Jordan A, Scholz R, Maier-Hauff K, van Landeghem FK, Waldoefner N, Teichgraeber U, Pinkernelle J, Bruhn H, Neumann F, Thiesen B, von Deimling A, Felix R. (2006) The effect of thermotherapy using magnetic nanoparticles on rat malignant glioma. *J Neurooncol* **78(1)**: 7-14.
85. Nirmal M and Brus LE. (1999) Luminescence photophysics in semiconductor nanocrystals. *Acc Chem Res* **32**: 407–414.
86. Dabbousi BO, Rodriguez-Viejo J, Mikulec FV, Heine JR, Mattoussi H, Ober R, Jensen KR, and Bawendi MG. (1997) (CdSe)ZnS Core-Shell Quantum Dots: Synthesis and Characterization of a Size Series of Highly Luminescent Nanocrystallites. *J Phys Chem B* **101(46)**: 9463-9475.
87. Lee LY, Ong SL, Hu JY, Ng WJ, Feng Y, Tan X, Wong SW. (2004) Use of semiconductor quantum dots for photostable immunofluorescence labeling of Cryptosporidium parvum. *Appl Environ Microbiol* **70(10)**: 5732-6.
88. Winter JO, Gomez N, Korgel BA, Schmidt CE. (2005) Quantum dots for electrical stimulation of neural cells. In: *Proceedings of SPIE: Nanobiophotonics and Biomedical Applications II* Cartwright AN and Osinski M (eds.) 5705: 235-246.
89. http://www.nidcd.nih.gov/health/hearing/coch.asp
90. http://www.neurophys.wisc.edu/h&b/textbook/chap-6.html

91. Leal MC, Shin YJ, Laborde ML, Calmels MN, Verges S, Lugardon S, Andrieu S, Deguine O, Fraysse B. (2003) Music perception in adult cochlear implant recipients. *Acta Otolaryngol* **23(7)**: 826-35.
92. White RD, Grosh K. (2005) Microengineered hydromechanical cochlear model. *Proc Natl Acad Sci U S A* **102(5)**: 1296-301.
93. http://news.bbc.co.uk/1/hi/health/4356266.stm
94. Schmidt EM, Bak MJ, Hambrecht FT, Kufta CV, O'Rourke DK, Vallabhanath P. Feasibility of a visual prosthesis for the blind based on intracortical microstimulation of the visual cortex. Brain. 1996 Apr; 119 (Pt 2): 507-22.
95. Normann RA, Warren DJ, Ammermuller J, Fernandez E, Guillory S. (2001) High-resolution spatio-temporal mapping of visual pathways using multi-electrode arrays. *Vision Res* **41(10-11)**: 1261-75.
96. Palanker D, Vankov A, Huie P, Baccus S. (2005) Design of a high-resolution optoelectronic retinal prosthesis. *J Neural Eng* **2(1)**: S105-20.
97. Veraart C, Wanet-Defalque MC, Gerard B, Vanlierde A, Delbeke J. (2003) Pattern recognition with the optic nerve visual prosthesis. *Artif Organs* **27(11)**: 996-1004.
98. Hochberg LR, Serruya MD, Friehs GM, Mukand JA, Saleh M, Caplan AH, Branner A, Chen D, Penn RD, Donoghue JP. (2006) Neuronal ensemble control of prosthetic devices by a human with tetraplegia. *Nature* **442(7099)**: 164-71.
99. Kennedy PR, Bakay RA. (1998) Restoration of neural output from a paralyzed patient by a direct brain connection. *Neuroreport* **9(8)**: 1707-11.
100. Kim HK, Biggs SJ, Schloerb DW, Carmena JM, Lebedev MA, Nicolelis MA, Srinivasan MA. (2006) Continuous shared control for stabilizing reaching and grasping with brain-machine interfaces. *IEEE Trans Biomed Eng* **53(6)**: 1164-73.
101. http://feswww.fes.cwru.edu/info/guide.php
102. Pfurtscheller G, Muller GR, Pfurtscheller J, Gerner HJ, Rupp R. (2003) 'Thought'--control of functional electrical stimulation to restore hand grasp in a patient with tetraplegia. *Neurosci Lett* **351(1)**: 33-6.
103. Elger CE, Lehnertz K. (1998) Seizure prediction by non-linear time series analysis of brain electrical activity. Eur J Neurosci **10(2)**: 786-9.
104. Zabara J. (1992) Inhibition of experimental seizures in canines by repetitive vagal stimulation. *Epilepsia* **33(6)**: 1005-12.
105. Borgens RB, Toombs JP, Breur G, Widmer WR, Waters D, Harbath AM, March P, Adams LG. (1999) An imposed oscillating electrical field improves the recovery of function in neurologically complete paraplegic dogs. *J Neurotrauma* **16(7)**: 639-57.
106. Rizzo JF 3rd, Wyatt J, Loewenstein J, Kelly S, Shire D. (2003) Perceptual efficacy of electrical stimulation of human retina with a microelectrode array during short-term surgical trials. *Invest Ophthalmol Vis Sci* **44**: 5362-9.
107. Griffith RW, Humphrey DR. (2007) Long-term gliosis around chronically implanted platinum electrodes in the Rhesus macaque motor cortex. *Neurosci Lett* Epub ahead of print.

108. Biran R, Martin DC, Tresco PA. (2005) Neuronal cell loss accompanies the brain tissue response to chronically implanted silicon microelectrode arrays. *Exp Neurol* **195(1)**: 115-26.
109. An KH, Jeon KK, Kim WS, Park YS, Lim SC, Bae DJ and Lee YH. (2001) Characterization of supercapacitors using singlewalled carbon nanotube electrodes. *J Korean Phys Soc* **39**: S511_S517.
110. Kim YH, Park CJ and Chang KJ. (2000) Sub-bands in carbon nanotubes under radial deformation. *J Korean Phys Soc* **37**: 85.
111. Wei J and Hong JB. (2000) Quasi-one dimensional model of carbon nanotubes. *J Korean Phys Soc* **38**: 602.
112. Chen C, Yan L, Kong S and Zhang Y. (2006) Ultrasonic nanowelding of carbon nanotubes to metal electrodes. *Nanotechology* **17 (9)**: 2192-2197.
113. http://www.sciencewatch.com/july-aug2004/sw_july-aug2004_page7.htm
114. Moxon KA, Kalkhoran NM, Markert M, Sambito MA, McKenzie JL, Webster TJ. (2004) Nanostructured surface modification of ceramic-based microelectrodes to enhance biocompatibility for a direct brain-machine interface. *IEEE Trans Biomed Eng* **51(6)**: 881-889.
115. Liopo AV, Stewart MP, Hudson J, Tour JM, Pappas TC. (2006) Biocompatibility of native and functionalized single-walled carbon nanotubes for neuronal interface. *J Nanosci Nanotechnol* **6(5)**: 1365-74.
116. Cambon K, Hansen SM, Venero C, Herrero AI, Skibo G, Berezin V, Bock E, Sandi C. (2004) A synthetic neural cell adhesion molecule mimetic peptide promotes synaptogenesis, enhances presynaptic function, and facilitates memory consolidation. *J Neurosci* **24(17)**: 4197-204.
117. Balazsi AG, Rootman J, Drance SM, Schulzer M, Douglas GR. (1984) The effect of age on the nerve fiber population of the human optic nerve. *Am J Ophthalmol* **97(6)**: 760-6.
118. Hebb DO. (1949) *The Organization of Behaviour: A Neuropsychological Theory*. Wiley, New York.
119. Mahadevappa M, Weiland JD, Yanai D, Fine I, Greenberg RJ, Humayun MS. (2005) Perceptual thresholds and electrode impedance in three retinal prosthesis subjects. *IEEE Trans Neural Syst Rehabil Eng* **13(2)**: 201-6.
120. http://oemagazine.com/fromTheMagazine/jul02/eyeontech.html
121. Sandison ME, Cooper JM. (2006) Nanofabrication of electrode arrays by electron-beam and nanoimprint lithographies. *Lab Chip* **6(8)**: 1020-5.
122. Kotwal A, Schmidt CE. (2001) Electrical stimulation alters protein adsorption and nerve cell interactions with electrically conducting biomaterials. *Biomaterials* **22(10)**: 1055-64.
123. http://www.physorg.com/news1361.html

124. Endo M, Hayashi T, Kim YA, Terrones M, Dresselhaus MS. (2004) Applications of carbon nanotubes in the twenty-first century. *Philos Transact A Math Phys Eng Sci* **362(1823)**: 2223-38.
125. http://pesn.com/2006/02/09/9600232_MIT_Battery/

Chapter 6

Vascular Nano Stents

Karen M. Haberstroh

1. Physiology of the Vascular System

The cardiovascular system is the transport system of the human body; it delivers nutrients and oxygen to cells of all tissue types while also removing waste products. This system consists of the heart, blood, and blood vessels, which act as the transport system pump, transport medium, and delivery routes, respectively.[1] Within the delivery route of the blood vessels are arteries, capillaries, and veins.[1] Briefly, the heart pumps oxygenated blood into the arteries, which become successively smaller as they feed into capillaries. Nutrients and gases are exchanged between blood and other tissues at the level of the capillaries. Blood is then fed into the veins, which carry de-oxygenated blood back to the heart.

1.1. Structure and Function of the Arterial System

Arteries are relatively thick as compared to the veins and capillaries; this is because their walls must be resilient enough to withstand the alternating pressures created by the pumping action of the heart. In addition, arterial walls possess unique viscoelastic mechanical properties which allow them to stretch when receiving an increased volume of blood, while also passively recoil when blood flows off into the circulation.

1.2. Components of the Artery Wall

The arterial wall features three layers: the intima, the media, and the adventitia (Fig. 1).[1,2] These layers encircle an inner cavity of the vessel known as the lumen, where blood flows.

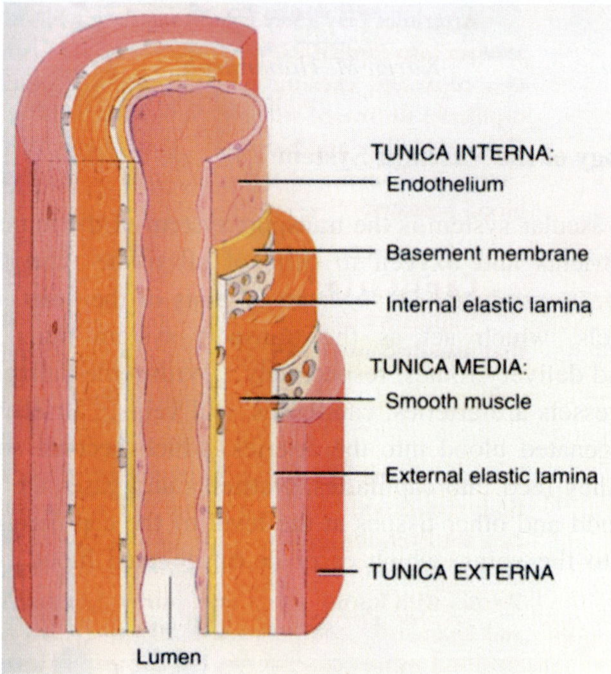

Figure 1. Blood vessel structure. [Adapted from[3]]

The intima is the innermost layer of the arterial wall; it directly surrounds the lumen. It is a thin layer composed of a monolayer of endothelial cells that fit tightly together. This monolayer of cells known as the endothelium creates a smooth lining capable of minimizing resistance to blood flow through the lumen.[1] The endothelium is supported by an extracellular matrix known as the basement membrane.[2]

The media is the thickest layer, from which arteries obtain most of their strength and resilience. This middle layer extends from the internal elastic lamina to the external elastic lamina and is composed of smooth muscle cells embedded in an extracellular matrix of elastin and collagen.[1,2] Smooth muscle cells contained within the media are oriented circumferentially and regulate the diameter of the vessel. Finally, the adventitia is the outermost layer of the arterial wall. It is composed primarily of fibrous connective tissue whose basic function is to provide support and protection to the vessel. [1]

1.3. Cells of the Vascular System

1.3.1. Vascular Endothelial Cells

Endothelial cells are thin, elongated cells that form a highly selective yet permeable barrier between blood elements and the underlying arterial wall. They consist of prominent nucleoli, many mitochondria, extensive endoplasmic reticulum and Golgi apparatus, many pinocytotic vesicles, and peripheral cytoplasmic microfilaments.[4] Endothelial cells grow in a monolayer, display a cobblestone morphology, and exhibit contact inhibition; this suggests that cells at the margins of an injury participate in repair processes.[4,5] Also, endothelial cells rest on a basement membrane made primarily of type IV collagen.[4] Endothelial cell functions ensure normal arterial blood flow and vessel wall hemeostasis.[4] Namely, these cells undergo drastic functional and structural modifications in response to various physopathological stimuli.[5] For example, endothelial cells are able to maintain a non thrombogenic surface in the vascular system by their production of compounds that inhibit platelet aggregation. They also have the ability to secrete procoagulant materials when needed.[4] Endothelial cells produce substances that control vessel tone including nitric oxide (NO, arguably the most important constriction and dilation factor in blood vessels). Finally, endothelial cells possess a variety of cell surface receptors, including those specific to inflammatory cells, low density lipoprotein (LDL), growth factors, inflammatory mediators, and a variety of pharmacologic agents.[4] As related to vessel dysfunction, injury to the endothelial layer is involved in the initiation of intimal lesion formation. This is because the presence or absence of an intact endothelium regulates proliferation of the underlying smooth muscle cells.[4,5] Under healthy conditions, the endothelium's inhibitory effect is likely due to either its selectively permeable barrier properties or its production of growth inhibitors; for example, heparin is synthesized by endothelial cells and is inhibitory to smooth muscle cells.[4]

1.3.2. Vascular Smooth Muscle Cells

Vascular smooth muscle cells are mainly found in the media of the arterial wall and modulate blood vessel functions by altering vascular wall tone in response to physiological changes, neural stimuli, and pharmacological interventions.[4] They synthesize and secret several forms of collagen, elastic proteins, and several types of proteoglycans. They possess a basal lamina which surrounds individual cell membranes; this is a characteristic feature of smooth muscle cells.[4] Smooth muscle cells exist in two different phenotypic forms: contractile and synthetic. The contractile phenotype is exhibited by resting vascular smooth muscle cells. In this form, smooth muscle cells are spindle shaped and have a single, elongated nucleus. These cells contain extensive cytoplasmic filaments but fewer mitochondria and endoplasmic reticulum; importantly, they do not readily respond to mitogens.[4] On the other hand, the synthetic phenotype is characteristic of proliferating smooth muscle cells; these cells have fewer contractile filaments, do not have the ability to contract, have an increased number of synthetic organelles, and produce numerous secretory proteins. Smooth muscle cells in the synthetic form are more responsive to mitogens.[4] Smooth muscle cells are key players in vascular disease and repair; in fact, they are the predominant constituents of intimal atherosclerotic lesions.[4]

1.3.3. Vascular Fibroblasts

Fibroblasts are spindly shaped cells that are present in all connective tissues. Their function is to synthesize collagen and other matrix materials. In the normal wound healing response, fibroblasts synthesize proteins (specifically, collagen and proteoglycans) that are part of the natural repair process. This process can lead down two different paths: fibrous encapsulation or regeneration. When fibrous encapsulation occurs, the body walls off the offending material in an effort to isolate it from the rest of the nearby tissue; the resulting scar tissue is usually non-functional. A more favorable reaction is tissue regeneration. During this process the granulation tissue is remodeled by parenchymal cells into native tissue that retains its function. In the case of vascular tissue, this would include a viable endothelial cell lining and smooth muscle cell layers.

1.3.4. Blood Cells

In addition to the major cell types found within the vessels themselves, blood is a connective tissue that consists of living cells suspended in a nonliving fluid matrix called the plasma.[1] Three main cells types are found in blood: red blood cells (erythrocytes) which transport oxygen, white blood cells (leukocytes) which are part of the body's immune system, and platelets which form blood clots (hemostasis).

2. Atherosclerosis: A Cardiovascular Disease

Cardiovascular diseases (or ailments of the heart and blood vessels) are the most common cause of death in the developed world. In the United States alone, more than 2,600 Americans die each day from cardiovascular disease.[2] More specifically, atherosclerosis is the underlying cause of about 50% of all deaths in the western world.[6,7] Atherosclerosis of the coronary artery accounts for most of those deaths, with more than 12 million Americans suffering from coronary artery disease.[2] Atherosclerosis is a diseased state of the middle- to large-sized arteries, in which the arterial wall hardens and thickens, leaving the lumen of the artery narrow. This stenosis is the result of plaque build-up in the lumen of the vessel, which slowly and silently progresses during a patient's lifetime (Fig. 2).

Over time, these changes result in obstruction of blood flow. For example, the vessel surface may become rough as a plaque protrudes into the blood, which leads to thrombus formation and further blocks blood flow. In addition, a reduced luminal area results in increased blood velocity through the diseased vessel. Furthermore, atherosclerotic vessels

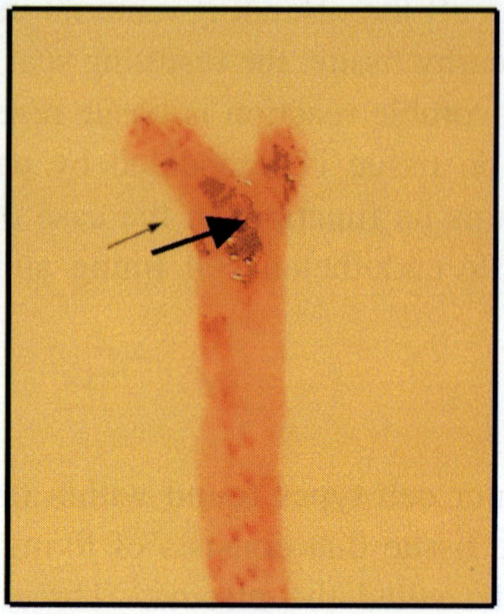

Figure 2. Lipid-rich atherosclerotic lesions present in the aortic arch of a Watanabe heritable hyperlipidemic rabbit.[8]

lose their distensibility and are easily ruptured. Factors such as injury, hemodynamic stress, lipoprotein metabolism, thrombosis, and inflammation may all play a role in the pathogenesis of this disease. Furthermore, other causative agents include hypertension, smoking, hyperlipidemia, homocystinemia, and diabetes mellitus.[9]

2.1. The Cellular Progression of Atherosclerosis

Endothelial cell dysfunction is characteristic of diseased vessels, including those plagued by atherosclerosis. This injury to the endothelial cell layer can range from cell denudation to alterations in normal cell functions.[4] For example, while endothelial cells normally participate in lipid uptake, this process is enhanced in the diseased state, thus resulting in the initiation of lesion (and thus plaque) formation. In addition, injured endothelial cells decrease their production of nitric oxide, which leads to impaired vasodilation and increased systemic blood pressure. Smooth muscle cells also play a role in this developing atherosclerotic plaque. Namely, they become activated by growth factors and cytokines released by a variety of vascular and blood borne cells. This leads to smooth muscle cell secretion of extracellular matrix components; at the same time, these cells proliferate at increased rates, migrate into the vessel lumen, and express altered genes.[10] Importantly, these released extracellular matrix components make up the fibrous cap of the atherosclerotic plaque. While it is now commonly accepted that vascular endothelial and smooth muscle cells are key components of disease development and progression, these cells do not act alone. Rather, atherosclerosis is critically affected by the role of monocytes and other inflammatory cell types. For instance, injured endothelial cells express selectins on their surface, thus, leading to a 'sticky' vessel wall. This mediates rolling and attachment of inflammatory cells along the endothelial cell layer, where they are able to migrate between the endothelial layer and into the intima.[10,12]

These monocytes then differentiate into macrophages – the major source of foam cells and the most predominant cell in the plaque.[10,11] Furthermore, they secrete biologically active products like IL-1 which affect endothelial and smooth muscle cell function.[10]

3. Treatments for Vascular Disease

The first step in treating diagnosed atherosclerosis is through medicine, diet, and exercise. However, when atherosclerosis and its resulting vessel occlusion progress to clinically noticeable and life-threatening levels, invasive medical interventions aimed at reopening the blocked artery must be considered.[7] In the most severe cases, this has been accomplished through bypass surgery, where a blood vessel is grafted at the diseased site to redirect blood flow around the occluded section of the artery. Although effective, this can be a dangerous procedure. Other therapies used in less severe cases include balloon angioplasty and stenting; each will be discussed in further detail in the sections that follow.

3.1. Balloon Angioplasty

More recent advances in the field have introduced angioplasty procedures for cases that are not as severe; more than 800,000 angioplasty procedures are performed in the United States alone each year.[2] Balloon angioplasty is appealing since it does not carry the risks associated with open-heart surgery.

Instead, a balloon-tipped catheter is fed to the diseased site; this balloon is inflated to reopen the artery by pushing the blockage against the walls of the artery and away from the lumen (Fig. 3). Despite the many benefits of treating coronary artery disease with angioplasty, a major drawback is restenosis, or re-narrowing of the lumen. Restenosis is different from the initial atherosclerotic lesion, becomes critical when the vessel lumen narrows by more than 50%, and usually calls for repeated invasive revascularization procedures.[2]

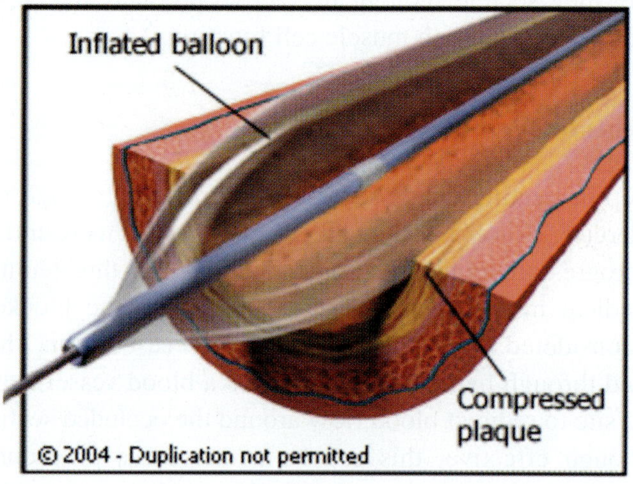

Figure 3. Schematic drawing of the balloon angioplasty procedure.[13]

Restenosis after angioplasty is caused by elastic recoil of the vessel, constrictive vascular remodeling, and smooth muscle cell proliferation with excessive extracellular matrix production at the site of injury.[2,14] Unfortunately, such restenosis is an irreversible process; hence all therapeutic approaches aimed at limiting restenosis are considered before, at the time of, or immediately after revascularization procedures.[2] Many therapeutic approaches have been proposed, including the use of drugs to inhibit the proliferation of smooth muscle cells. Two such drugs that have potential in the field are rapamycin (Sirolimus) and pactlitaxel (Taxol), which have been shown to inhibit neointimal proliferation.[2,15] However, since these drugs may have potentially dangerous side-effects, stent implantation is the first and most effective means of reducing restenosis after angioplasty. [2,14,15]

3.2. Vascular Stents

In an effort to reduce restenosis rates, balloon angioplasty is often followed by insertion of a reinforcement stent. In this procedure, a hollow metal wire mesh tube (the stent) is inserted at the diseased site to push and hold the blockage against the artery walls and away from the lumen (Fig. 4). Stents are made of metals such as stainless steel, titanium and nickel alloys.[16] Recently, alloys of cobalt chromium have also found prominence in the field.[17,18] The most important basis for choosing a metal for stent applications is biocompatibility.[16]

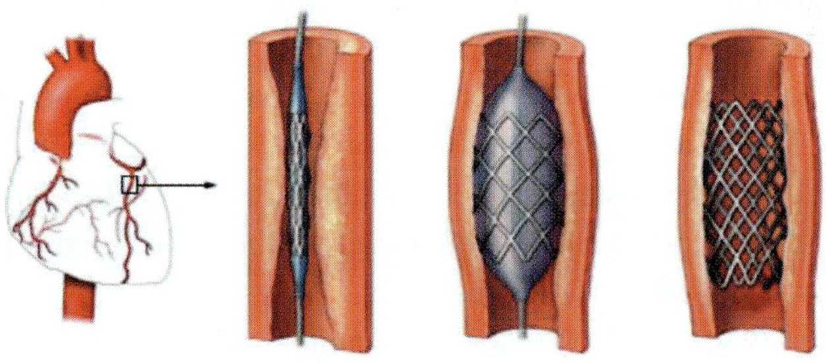

Figure 4. Insertion of metal stent using a balloon inflated device.[19]

Titanium and cobalt chromium alloys are most biocompatible because they are corrosion resistant in the body – specifically, in vivo, titanium forms an inert titanium oxide layer on the surface of the metal.[20]

In contrast, stainless steel is the least corrosion resistant.[16] Nitinol (nickel-titanium alloy) has also received recent attention since it would provide stents with desirable shape memory properties; however the high amounts of nickel have limited the use of nitinol in stent applications (note that large amounts of nickel can be cytotoxic and carcinogenic).[20] Therefore, researchers have proposed to use nitinol solely as a base stent material; modifying the nitinol surface by oxidizing heat treatment would form a cytocompatible layer of titanium oxide on its surface.[20]

3.2.1. The Use of Nano-structured Biomaterials in Vascular Stent Applications

In an effort to further enhance cell biocompatibility to biomaterials, many researchers have investigated the use of a novel class of materials with nano-structured surface features (or surface features less than 100nm in size). This approach has been taken in an effort to better mimic the natural architecture of the host tissue and its extracellular matrix, which also possess nano-structured features. For example, Goodman et al. created a polymethylmethacrylate (PMMA) mold of a denuded canine artery (Fig. 5) which clearly depicts the unique heterogeneous nano-structured features present in vascular tissue.[21]

Not surprisingly, such nano surface roughness has been shown to influence protein adsorption and subsequent cellular responses. Specifically, previous in vitro results have provided evidence that polymers with nano-dimensional surface features enhanced bladder smooth muscle cell adhesion, proliferation, and the production of critical extracellular matrix proteins.[22-24] This trend also held for vascular endothelial and smooth muscle cells tested on the similar nano-structured PLGA films.[25] Furthermore, ceramics, polymers, and metals (like titanium, Ti6Al4V, and CoCrMo) with nano-structured surface features enhanced osteoblast and chondrocyte functions.[27-29] More recently, research has been conducted to determine the potential role of nano-structured materials in vascular stent applications. Specifically, Choudhary et al. investigated vascular endothelial and smooth muscle cell adhesion on nano- structured compared to conventional titanium; these nano-structured surfaces had a greater root mean squared surface

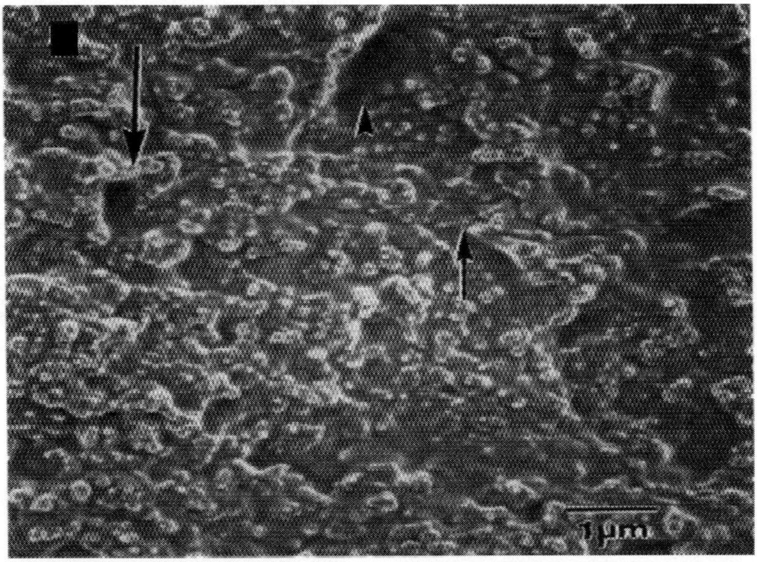

Figure 5. Mold of a denuded canine artery, which clearly depicts nano-structured features present in vascular tissue. Scale bar = 1 μm. Arrows indicate numerous nanometer features.[21]

roughness as characterized by SEM images (Fig. 6A) and as quantified using AFM technologies.[29] Results of their study confirmed increased vascular cell adhesion, along with a more well-spread cell morphology, on nano-structured compared to conventional titanium after 4 hours (Fig. 6B). Such coverage of the luminal surface of a vascular stent by endothelial cells implies a greater protection of the underlying metal surface to detrimental interactions with blood cells. Moreover, data suggested that the ratio of endothelial to vascular smooth muscle cells slightly increased on nano-structured compared to conventional titanium. This is significant since a major mode of stent failure involves the attachment of greater numbers of vascular smooth muscle cells as compared to endothelial cells in the vascular lumen.[30] In combination, these findings suggest that vascular stents composed of nanometer-sized particles may invoke advantageous cellular responses for vascular stent applications.

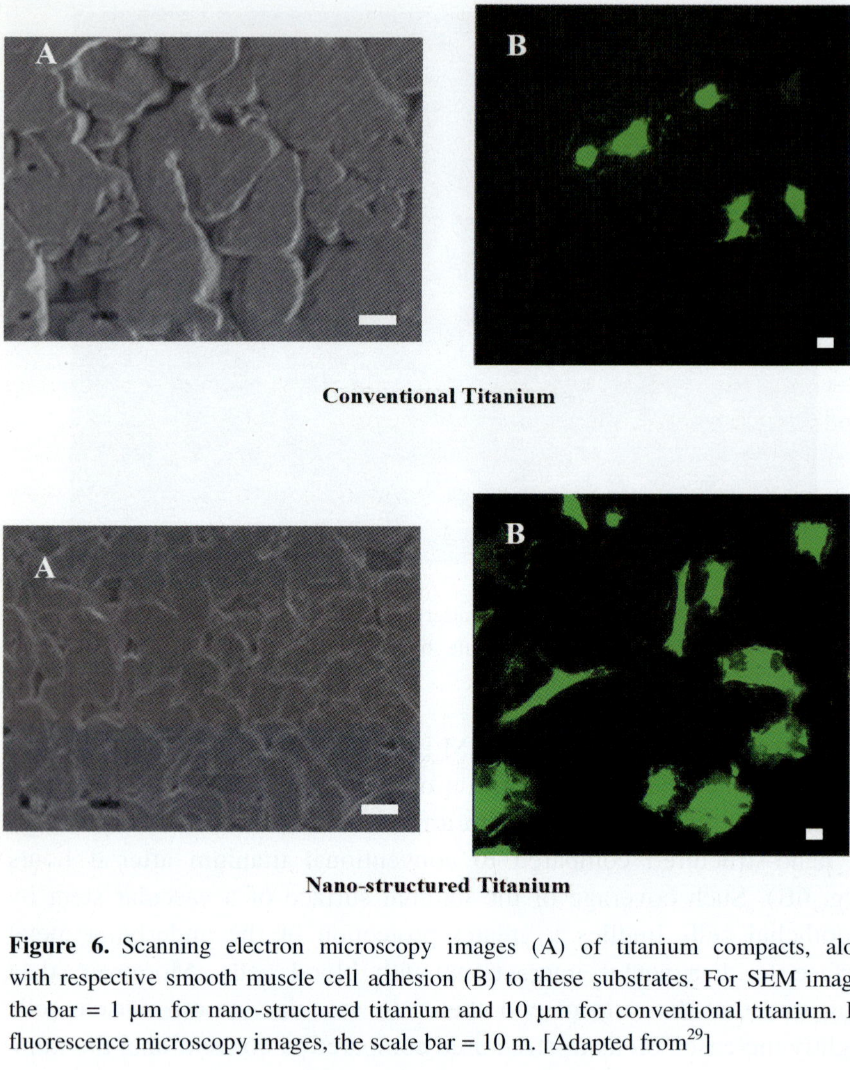

Figure 6. Scanning electron microscopy images (A) of titanium compacts, along with respective smooth muscle cell adhesion (B) to these substrates. For SEM images, the bar = 1 μm for nano-structured titanium and 10 μm for conventional titanium. For fluorescence microscopy images, the scale bar = 10 m. [Adapted from[29]]

3.2.2. Problems with Current Stent Designs

Regardless of the material used, it is important to note that stenting has been successful in reducing restenosis rates. It has not, however, been able to completely eliminate the problem; on average, restenosis still occurs in about 20% of patients undergoing the procedure.[2,15,31] In-stent restenosis is generally attributed to neointimal formation, or the proliferation of smooth muscle cells and production of extracellular matrix.[2] The degree of injury placed on the artery wall by the stent correlates with the extent of inflammation and neointimal formation.[2] A direct relationship also exists between the number of monocytes in the injured area and the extent of intimal growth, suggesting that the inflammatory reaction contributes to neointimal formation during in-stent restenosis.[2] Further aggravation of the vessel occurs due to the stresses and strains placed on the vascular wall when the stent is in place. Finally, the presence of the foreign material elicits the "foreign body response" and causes inflammation in an attempt to reject the material.

Drug-eluting stents have been used to counteract many of these issues. For example, rapamycin or paclitaxel have been coated on the stent and delivered directly to the site of injury in order to limit restenosis by inhibiting the proliferation of smooth muscle cells.[32] Since inflammation is also a major contributor to restenosis, the use of immunosuppressive drug-eluting stents has also provided promising results when considering restenosis treatment.[33] Unfortunately, drug eluting stents can not counteract a less recognized problem: namely, the formation of stent wear debris. This becomes especially critical when considering the repair of long or branched vessels.[34] These situations often require multiple stents, which may overlap. In this case, the metal stent surfaces may rub against one another due to the cyclic pulsing of the vasculature, or simply as the result of bodily movements. If this were to occur, it would undoubtedly yield wear particles in the vicinity of the stent or even elsewhere in the body.

3.2.3. Stent Wear Debris

To date, few studies have considered the potential role that stent wear debris may play in normal tissue function. One study did investigate the in situ surface wear properties of surface modified nickel titanium shape memory alloy as proposed for use in vascular applications.[34] Namely, materials in the both the austenitic and martensitic form were tested using a stainless steel counter wearing surface, at a load of 0.2N and at a frequency of 20Hz for 10,000 cycles. Results provided evidence of Ni-Ti high wear resistance, which was attributed to its ability to undergo pseudoelastic transformation under loading. Other factors affecting the extent of wear included surface hardness, contact stress, relative motion of the wearing bodies, lubricant, and temperature.[34] Although this study provided useful information with regards to a very promising material (Ni-Ti shape memory alloy) for stent applications, it has not begun to test the in vitro or in vivo biocompatibility or cytotoxicity of these same materials with vascular cells. This is critical as even very small amounts of wear debris/particles may adversely affect vascular cell (and thus tissue) functions. Another organ system which has been more widely studied with respect to detrimental metal and ceramic wear properties is bone. Namely, wear particles can induce bone loss, thus leading to implant loosening and eventual long-term failure of joint replacements.[35-41] To date, in vitro studies have primarily focused on understanding the role of micron-sized particles on bone cell function.[42-49]

In addition, more recent studies have suggested that materials made of nano-sized particles (and thus, with nano- particulate wear debris) may enhance cell viability. This has indeed been shown for both chondrocytes and osteoblasts (the bone forming cells). For example, after 2 hours and compared to conventional (micron sized) titania particles, osteoblasts exhibited significantly greater numbers in the presence of nano particulates.[50] Interestingly, viable cells also maintained the well-spread morphology characteristic of healthy bone cells (Fig. 7); in fact, nano particulates appeared to be simply "engulfed" by the cell (Fig. 7) as opposed to the case of the micron sized particles which appeared to surround and crowd out the cell body (Fig. 7).[50]

Although not studied to date, this study suggests that metals fabricated to possess nano- structured surface features may reduce many of the negative consequences of vascular wear debris.

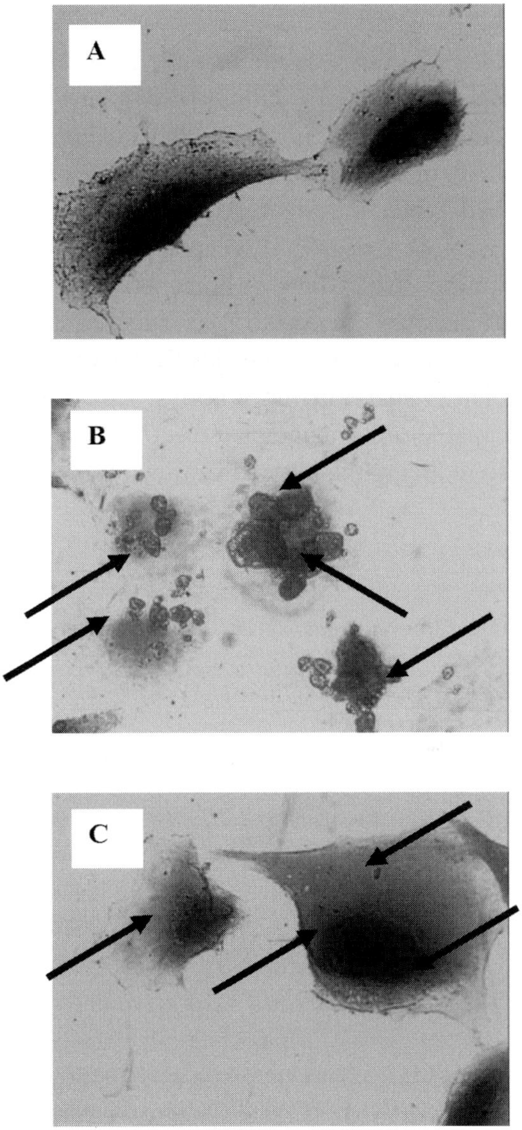

Figure 7. Osteoblasts in the presence of no particulates (control; A), conventional alumina particles (B), and nanophase alumina particles (C) for 2 hours. [Adapted from[50]]

4. Conclusions

In summary, vascular stenting procedures have been fairly successful in reducing restenosis associated with atherosclerosis and balloon angioplasty. In-stent restenosis is generally attributed to neointimal formation, aggravation of the vessel due to the stresses and strains placed on the vascular wall when the stent is in place, the presence of the foreign material (i.e., the "foreign body response"), and the formation of stent wear debris (in the case of long or branched vessels). Based on this knowledge, further improvements to the success rates of stenting procedures may be achieved with the development of novel material formulations (like Ni-TI shape memory alloys, nano- structured metals, etc), which are capable of enhancing select cell functions to those materials while also reducing the toxicity of inevitable wear particles.

Bibliography

1. Marieb EN. (2001) *Human Anatomy & Physiology 5th Edition*, Benjamin Cummings, New York.
2. Marschall SR and Patterson C. (2005) *Principles of Molecular Cardiology*, Humana Press, New Jersey.
3. Tortora GJ and Grabowksi SR. (2000) *Principles of Anatomy and Physiology 9th Edition*, John Wiley and Sons, New York.
4. White RA. (1989) *Atherosclerosis and Arteriosclerosis*, CRC Press, Florida.
5. Simionescu N and Simionescu M. *Endothelial Cell Dysfunction*, Plenum Press, New York and London.
6. Lusis AJ. (2000) Artherosclerosis *Nature* **407**: 233-241 (2000).
7. Hoffman GS and Weyand CM. (2002) *Inflammatory Diseases of Blood Vessel*, Marcel Dekker, New York.
8. Topper JN and Gimbrone MA Jr. (1999) Artherosclerosis. *Molecular Medicine Today* **5**: 40-46.
9. White RA and Hollier LH. (2005) *Vascular Surgery: Basic Science and Clinical Correlations 2nd Edition*, Blackwell Publishing, Massachusetts.
10. Hansson GK. (2001) Drug eluting stents. *Arterioscler Thromb Vasc Biol* **21(12)**: 1876-90.
11. Robenek H and Severs NJ. (1992) *Cell Interactions in Atherosclerosis* CRC Press, Boca Raton.
12. Blake GJ and Ridker PM. (2001). Metal stents *Circ Res* **89(9)**: 763-71.
13. Heart Center Online at www.heartcenteronline.com

14. Linde J and Strauss BH. (2001) Pharmacological treatment for prevention of restenosis *Expert Opin Emerg Drugs* **6(2)**: 281-302.
15. van der Hoeven BL, Pires NM, Warda HM, Oemrawsingh PV, van Vlijmen BJ, Quax PH, Schalij MJ, van der Wall EE, and Jukema JW. (2005) Drug eluting stents: results, promises, problems. *Int J Cardiol* **99**: 9-17.
16. Gotman I. (1997) Characteristics of metals used in implants. *J Endourol* **11**: 383-9
17. Kereiakes DJ, Cox DA, Hermiller JB, Midei MG, Bachinsky WB, Nukta ED, Leon MB, Fink S, Marin L, and Lansky AJ. (2003) Usefulness of a cobalt chromium coronary stent alloy. *Am J Cardiol* **92(4)**: 463-6.
18. Sketch MH Jr, Ball M, Rutherford B, Popma JJ, Russell C, and Kereiakes DJ. (2005) Evaluation of the Medtronic (Driver) cobalt-chromium alloy coronary stent system. *Am J Cardiol* **95(1)**: 8-12.
19. University Health Systems of Eastern Carolina at www.uhseast.com
20. Plant SD, Grant DM, and Leach L. (2005) Behaviour of human endothelial cells on surface modified NiTi alloy..*Biomaterials* **26(26)**: 5359-67.
21. Goodman SL, Sims PA, and Albrecht RM. (1996) Mimicking the roughness of vascular tissue. *Biomaterials* **17(21)**: 2087-95.
22. Thapa A, Webster TJ, and Haberstroh KM. (2003) Polymers with nano-dimensional surface features enhance bladder smooth muscle cell adhesion. *Journal of Biomedical Materials Research* **67A(4)**: 1374-83.
23. Thapa A, Miller DC, Webster TJ, and Haberstroh KM. (2003) Nano-structured polymers enhance bladder smooth muscle cell function. *Biomaterials* **24(17)**: 2915-2926.
24. Pattison MA, Webster TJ, Wurster S, and Haberstroh KM. (2005) Three-dimensional, nano-structured PLGA scaffolds for bladder tissue replacement applications *Biomaterials* **26(15)**: 2491-500.
25. Miller DC, Thapa A, Haberstroh KM, and Webster TJ. (2004) Mechanisms of increased vascular cell adhesion on nanostructured poly(lactic-co-glycolic acid) films. *Biomaterials* **25(1)**: 53-61.
26. Webster TJ, Ergun C, Doremus RH, Siegel RW, and Bizios R. (2000) Enhanced functions of osteoblasts on nanophase ceramics. *Biomaterials*.**21(17)**: 1803-10.
27. Webster TJ and Ejiofor JU. (2004) Increased osteoblast adhesion on nanophase metals: Ti, Ti6Al4V, and CoCrMo. *Biomaterials* **25(19)**: 4731-9.
28. Park GE, Pattison MA, Park K, and Webster TJ. (2005) Accelerated chondrocyte functions on NaOH-treated PLGA scaffolds. *Biomaterials* **26(16)**: 3075-82.
29. Choudhary S, Berhe M, Haberstroh KM, and Webster TJ. (2006). Increased vascular cell adhesion on nanostructured metals. *International Journal of Nanotechnology* **1(1)**: 41-49.
30. Messer RL, Wataha JC, Lewis JB, Lockwood PE, Caughman GB, and Tseng WY. (2005) Metal stents. *J Long-term Effects of Medical Implants* **15(1)**: 39-47.
31. Huang Y, Salu K, Wang L, Liu X, Li S, Lorenz G, Wnendt S, Verbeken E, Bosmans J, Van de Werf F, and De Scheerder I. (2005) Use of tacrolimus-eluting stent to

inhibit neointimal hyperplasia in a porcine coronary model. *J Invasive Cardiol* **17**: 142-148.

32. Moreno R and Macaya C. (2005) Stent-based delivered anti-proliferative drugs in the prevention of coronary stent restenosis. *Curr Med Chem Cardiovasc Hematol Agents* **3(3)**: 221-9.
33. Donners MM, Daemen MJ, Cleutjens KB, and Heeneman S. (2003) Inflammation and restenosis: implications for therapy. *Ann Med* **35**: 523-31.
34. Tan L, Crone WC, and Sridharan K. (2002) *J Mater Sci Mater Med* **13(5)**: 501-8.
35. Oparaugo PC, Clarke IC, Malchau H, and Herberts P. (2001) Correlation of wear debris-induced osteolysis and revision with volumetric wear-rated of polyethylene: a survey of 8 reports in the literature. *Acta Orthop Scand* **72**: 22–28.
36. Urban RM, Jacobs JJ, Tomlinson MJ, Gavrilovic J, Black J, and Peoc ' h M. (2000). Dissemination of wear particles to the liver, spleen, and abdominal lymph nodes of patients with hip or knee replacement. *J Bone Jt Surg Am* **82**: 457–476.
37. Hashiguchi T, Hirano T, Shindo H, and Baba K. (1999) Wear of alumina prosthesis. *Arch Orthop Trauma Surg* **119**: 30–34.
38. Kobayashi A, Bonfield W, Kadoya Y, Yamac T, Freeman MA, Scott G, and Revell PA. (1997) The size and shape of particulate polyethylene wear debris in total joint replacements. *Proceedings of the Institution of Mechanical Engineering Part H - J Eng Med* **211**: 11–15.
39. Lerouge S, Huk O, Yahia LH, and Sedel L. (1996) Characterization of in vivo wear debris from ceramic-ceramic total hip arthroplasties. *J Biomed Mater Res* **32**: 627–633.
40. Savio JA III, Overcamp LM, and Black J. (1994) Size and shape of biomaterial wear debris. *Clin Mater* **15**: 101–147.
41. Buly RL, Huo MH, Salvati E, Brein W, and Bansal M. (1992) Wear debris in failed cemented total hip arthroplasty. An analysis of 71 cases. *J. Arthroplasty* **7**: 315–323.
42. Schanbhag AS, Jacobs JJ, Black J, Galante JO, and Glant TT. (1997) Glant, Effects of particles on fibroblast proliferation and bone resorption in vitro. *Clin Orthop Relat Res* **342**: 205–217.
43. Green TR, Fisher J, Stone M, Wroblewski BM, and Ingham E. (1998) Polyethylene particles of a 'critical size' are necessary for the induction of cytokines by macrophages in vitro. *Biomaterials* **19**: 2297–2302.
44. Pioletti DP, Takei H, Kwon Sym Wood D, and Sung KL. (1999). The cytotoxic effect of titanium particles phagocytosed by osteoblasts. *J Biomed Mater Res* **46**: 399–407.
45. Kohilas K, Lyons M, Lofthouse R, Frondoza CG, Jinnah R, and Hungerford DS. (1999) Effect of prosthetic titanium wear debris on mitogen-induced monocyte and lymphoid activation. *J Biomed Mater Res* **47**: 95–103.
46. Lohmann CH, Schwartz Z, Koster G, Jahn U, Buchhorn GH, MacDougall MJ, Casasola D, Liu Y, Sylvia VL, Dean DD, and Boyan BD. (2000) Phagocytosis of

wear debris by osteoblasts affects differentiation and local factor production in a manner dependent on particle composition. *Biomaterials* **21**: 551–561.

47. Kwon SY, Takei H, Pioletti DP, Lin T, Ma QJ, Akeson WH, Wood DJ, and Sung KL. (2000) Titanium particles inhibit osteoblast adhesion to fibronectin-coated substrates. *J Orthop Res* **18**: 203–211.
48. DeHeer DH, Engles JA, DeVries AS, Knapp RH, and Beebe JD. (2001). In situ complement activation by polyethylene wear debris. *J Biomed Mater Res* **54**: 12–19.
49. Vermes C, Chandrasekaran R, Jacobs JJ, Galante JO, Roebuck KA, and Glant TT. (2001) The effects of particulate wear debris, cytokines, and growth factors on the functions of MG-63 osteoblasts. *J Bone Jt Surg Am* **83**: 201–211.
50. Gutwein LG and Webster TJ. (2004) Increased viable osteoblast density in the presence of nanophase compared to conventional alumina and titania particles *Biomaterials* **25(18)**: 4175-83.

Chapter 7

Nanoparticles: Determining Toxicity

Ezharul Hoque Chowdhury and Toshihiro Akaike

1. Introduction

Biocompatibility is defined as the ability of a material to exist alongside living systems without harming them. Assessment of biocompatibility is a measure of the magnitude and duration of the adverse alterations of biological responses initiated by a material. Since nanoparticles have the tremendous potentials for being extensively used especially in biomedical engineering for drug delivery, tissue remodeling and diagnosis, evaluation of their biocompatibility is an indispensable task considering their safety issue in human beings.[1] The ratio of surface to total atoms or molecules increases exponentially with decreasing particle size and this increased surface area enables nanoparticles to exhibit greater biological activity per given mass compared with larger particles in either a positive manner leading to beneficial therapeutic activities or an unexpected toxicity problem.

Since adverse health effects could result from exposure to the nanoparticle-based devices, preclinical assessment of the toxic potential of the nanoparticles is needed to minimize the potential hazard to the patient. At present, safety assessments of such medical devices are guided by the toxicological and other studies recommended in the International Organization for Standardization (ISO) standard. ISO is in the process of publishing a series of standards on the biological evaluation of medical devices—ISO 10993.[2] Many parts of this series have been accepted as international standards, while the rest are under development.[3] Tests that may be used in an evaluation of device biocompatibility include procedures for cytotoxicity, skin sensitization, dermal irritation and intracutaneous reactivity, acute systemic toxicity, subchronic toxicity, mutagenicity, implantation, hemocompatibility, chronic toxicity, carcinogenicity, reproductive and developmental toxicity, biodegradation and immune responses

2. Strategies for Biocompatibility Testing

2.1. Cytotoxicity

Cytotoxicity is a rapid, sensitive and inexpensive test to detect the potential ability of a device to induce sublethal or lethal effects observed at the cellular level. Three main types of cell-culture assays have been developed: the elution test, the direct-contact test, and the agar diffusion test as described by the ISO 10993-5 standard.[2] In the elution test, an extract of the material is prepared and added in varied concentrations to the cell cultures. Growth inhibition is a widely used parameter, but others may also be used. In the direct-contact test, pieces of test material are placed directly on top of the cell layer, which is covered only by a layer of liquid cell-culture medium. Toxic molecules which could be nano-size particles, leaching from the test material may depress the growth rate of the cells or damage them in various ways. In the agar diffusion test, a piece of test material is placed on an agar layer covering a confluent monolayer of cells. Toxic molecules leaching from the material diffuse through the thin agar layer and kill or disrupt adjacent cells in the monolayer. The physical and chemical properties of the test material should be considered before the choice of the test system is made.

There is usually a good qualitative correlation between results from cell-culture tests and studies performed in vivo with respect to cytotoxicity versus primary tissue effects. It is important to recognize, however, that although cell-culture toxicity is in general a good and sensitive indicator of primary tissue compatibility, exceptions may arise in cases where leaching substances cause tissue damage in vivo through more complex mechanisms. At present, the in vitro cytotoxicity assays should be used as screening tests and considered primarily as supplements to the various in vivo tests.

2.2. Sensitization, Irritation and Intracutaneous Reactivity

Exposure to or contact with even minute amounts of potential leachable agents or nanomaterials can result in allergic or sensitization reactions. Sensitization tests that estimate the potential for contact sensitization of devices, materials and/or their extracts are usually carried out in guinea pigs and should reflect the intended route (skin, eye, mucosa) and nature, degree, frequency, duration, and conditions of exposure of the biomaterials in its intended clinical use. The preferred animal species for skin irritation tests is the albino rabbit, whose highly sensitive, light skin makes it possible to detect even very slight skin irritation caused by a substance. Skin reaction is seen as redness or swelling and is graded according to a specified classification system. Dermal irritation is the production of reversible changes in the skin following the application of a substance, whereas dermal corrosion is the production of irreversible tissue damage (scar formation) in the skin. Materials that consist of corrosive substances are not likely candidates for medical device production. Intracutaneous (intradermal) reactivity tests determine the localized reaction of tissue to the extracts of medical devices, biomaterials or prostheses in the final product form. Undesirable intracutaneous reactivity includes redness or swelling.

2.3. Acute Systemic Toxicity

Acute systemic toxicity is the adverse effect occurring within a short time after administration of a single dose of a substance. ISO 10993-1 requires that the test for acute systemic toxicity be considered for all device categories that indicate blood contact. Materials or extracts of medical devices are usually administered intravenously or intraperitoneally in rabbits or mice. Determining acute systemic toxicity is usually an initial step in the assessment and evaluation of the toxic characteristics of a substance. By providing information on health hazards likely to arise from short-term exposure, the acute systemic toxicity test can serve as a first step in the establishment of a dosage regimen in subchronic and other studies, and can also supply initial data on the mode of toxic action of a substance.

2.4. Genotoxicity

Genetic toxicology tests can be used to investigate nanomaterials for possible mutagenic effects leading to damage to the body's genes or chromosomes. The tests are performed both in vitro and in vivo. In vivo genetoxicity tests are carried out if indicated by the chemistry and/or composition of the material or if in vitro test results indicate potential genetoxicity. The initial in vitro assays should cover the three levels of genotoxic effects: DNA effects, gene mutations and chromosomal-aberrations. In vivo genetoxicity tests include the micronucleus test, the in vivo mammalian bone marrow cytogenetic tests, chromosomal analysis, the rodent dominant lethal tests, the mammalian germ line cytogenic assay, the mouse spot test, and the mouse heritable translocation assay. Not all of the in vivo genotoxicity tests need to be performed, and the most common test is the rodent micronucleus test.

2.5. Implantation

Implantation tests are designed to assess any localized effects of a device used inside the human body. Implantation testing methods essentially attempt to imitate the intended use conditions of an implanted material. Although different tests use various animal species, the rabbit has become the species of choice, with implantation performed in the paravertebral muscle. Implantation can be either surgical or nonsurgical: the surgical method involves the creation of a pouch in the muscle into which the implant is placed, while the nonsurgical method uses a cannula and stylet to insert a cylinder-shaped implant. Through a macroscopic examination the degree of tissue reaction in the paravertebral muscle is evaluated as a measure of biocompatibility.

2.6. Hemacompatibility

Hemacompatibility tests can evaluate effects on blood and/or blood components by blood-contacting medical devices or nanomaterials. In vivo hemacompatibility tests are usually designed to simulate the geometry, contact conditions and flow dynamics of the device or materials in its clinical application. From the ISO standards perspective, five test categories are indicated for hemacompatibility evaluation: thrombosis, coagulation, platelets, hematology and immunology. Several issues are important in the selection of tests for hemacompatibility. While in vivo testing in animals may be convenient, species differences in blood reactivity must be considered.

2.7. Subchronic and Chronic Toxicity

Subchronic toxicity is the potentially adverse effect that can occur as a result of the repeated daily dosing of a substance or nanomaterials to experimental animals over a portion of their life span. In the assessment and evaluation of the toxic characteristics of a chemical, the determination of subchronic toxicity is carried out after initial information on toxicity has been obtained by acute testing, and provides data of possible health hazards likely to arise from repeated exposures over a limited time. Such testing can provide information about target organs and the possibilities of toxin accumulation, and provide an estimate of a no-effect exposure level that can be used to select dose levels for chronic studies and establish safety criteria for human exposure. In subchronic or chronic toxicity studies, one or two animal species are dosed daily, usually for a period of 3 to 6 months, the rat is the standard animal species of choice.

2.8. Carcinogenicity

The objective of long-term carcinogenicity studies is to observe experimental animals over a major portion of their life span to detect any development of neoplastic lesions (tumor induction) during or after exposure to various doses of a test substance or nanoparticles. Carcinogenicity tests should be conducted only if data from other sources suggest a tendency for tumor induction. Carcinogenicity testing is normally conducted with oral dosing. For implants and medical devices, however, only extracts can be tested and they must be administered intravenously. In carcinogenicity studies, mice or rats are dosed every day for 18 to 24 months. At the completion of the dosing period, all surviving animals are sacrificed and their organs and tissues are examined microscopically for the presence of tumors. An increased incidence of one or more category of tumors in the dosed group would indicate that the product tested has the potential to induce tumors and could be considered a possible carcinogen in humans.

2.9. Reproductive and Developmental Toxicity

These tests can evaluate the potential effects of medical devices, their extracts or nano-materials on reproductive function, embryonic development and prenatal and early postnatal development. The application site of the device must be considered and test and/or bioassays should only be conducted when the device has potential impact on the reproductive potential of the subject.

2.10. Biodegradation

Biodegradation tests determine the effects of a biodegradable nano-material and their products on the tissue response. Emphasis is given on the amount of degradation during a given period of time, the nature of the degradation products, the origin of the degradation products and the qualitative and quantitative assessment of degradation products and leachable agents in adjacent tissues and in distant organs.

2.11. Immune Responses

Immune response evaluation is not a component of the standards currently available for tissue compatibility assessment. However, government agencies, such as FDA (Food and Drug Administration) and regulatory bodies, such as ISO currently emphasize for immune response evaluation where pertinent.[4] An example of the need for immune response evaluation is with modified natural tissue implants, such as collagen, which has been utilized in a number of different types of implants. Viral particles which are extensively used for gene therapy research, is another example where adverse immunological reactions may occur. Immunotoxic effects occur when humoral or cellular immunity needed by the host to defend itself against infections, neoplastic disease or unnecessary tissue damage is compromised. Potential immunological effects that may be associated are hypersensitivity, chronic inflammation, immunosuppression, immunostimulation and autoimmunity.

3. Route of Entry and Biokinetics of Nanoparticles

Most of the research related to the assessment of nanoparticle biocompatibility has been carried out in mammalian systems, with a focus on respiratory system exposures. However, there are other exposures routes, such as skin or GI (gastrointestinal) tract that also need to be considered as potential portals of entry. Although route-specific defense mechanisms protect the mammalian organism from harmful materials, these defenses may not always be effective for nanoparticles.[5,6] Not only environmentally, but also internationally for therapeutic purpose, nanoparticles would be allowed to penetrate through the above routes and additionally directly in the blood circulation.

3.1. Respiratory Tract

There are significant differences between nanoparticles and larger particles regarding their behavior during deposition and clearance in the respiratory tract. The main mechanism for deposition of inhaled nanoparticles is diffusion due to displacement when they collide with air molecules. Electrostatic precipitation occurs only in cases where nanoparticles carry significant electric charges. Inhaled nanoparticles can target the nasopharyngeal, tracheobronchial and alveolar regions of the respiratory tract, Several defense mechanisms exist throughout the respiratory tract aimed at keeping the mucosal surfaces free from particles deposited by inhalation.[7,8] Once deposited, nanoparticles appear to translocate readily to extrapulmonary sites and reach other target organs by different transfer routes and mechanisms.

3.1.1. Alveolar Macrophage-Mediated Clearance

The most prevalent mechanism for solid particle clearance in the alveolar region is mediated by alveolar macrophages through phagocytosis of deposited particles. The success of macrophage-particle encounter appears to be facilitated by chemotactic attraction of alveOlar macrophages to the site of particle deposition.[9] The chemotactic signal is most likely complement protein 5a (C5a), derived from activation of the complement cascade from serum proteins present on the alveolar surface.[10, 11] This is followed by gradual movement of the macrophages with internalized particles toward the mucociliary escalator. The retention half-time of solid particles in the alveolar region based on this clearance mechanism is about 70 days in rats and up to 700 days in humans. The efficacy of this clearance mechanism depends highly on the efficiency of alveolar macrophages to sense deposited particles. This process of phagocytosis of all of the deposited particles takes place within 6-12 hr to facilitate the subsequent removal by the slow alveolar clearance mentioned above, it appears that there are significant particle-size dependent differences in the cascade of alveolar macrophage-mediated clearance. When rats were exposed to the different-sized polystyrene particles, approximately 80% of 0.5-, 3- and 10-μm particles could be retrieved with the macrophages, whereas only approximately 20% of nano-sized 15-20 nm and 80-nm particles could be retrieved with the macrophages.[12-14] This indicated that nanoparticles either were in epithelial cells or had further translocated to the interstitium.

3.1.2. Translocation across Epithelial and Endothelial Cell Layers

Because of the apparent inefficiency of alveolar macrophage phagocytosis of nanoparticles, it appears that there could be other route of nanoparticle translocation. Indeed, results from some studies using ultrafine PTFE fumes and TiO_2 nanoparticles, show that nanoparticles deposited, readily gain access to interstitial sites through transcytosis across epithelia of the respiratory tract.[13,15,16] Because such translocation of fine particles across the alveolar epithelium is more prominent in larger species (dogs, non-human primates) than in rodents, it is reasonable to assume that the high translocation of nanoparticles occurs in human as well.[6,17] Once the particles reach pulmonary interstitial sites, uptake into the blood circulation, in addition to lymphatic pathways, can occur. Using intratracheal instillations of 30-nm gold particles in rats, it was found that within 30 min post-exposure large amount of the particles accumulated in platelets of pulmonary capillaries.[18] This translocation across epithelial and endothelial cell layers is governed by particle size, surface chemistry (coating) and possibly charge.[19,20] Albumin, the most abundant protein in plasma and interstitium, appears to facilitate nanoparticle endocytosis, as does lecithin, a phospholipids. The 240 nm polystyrene particles even translocated across the alveolo-capillary barrier when coated with lecithin, whereas uncoated particles did not.[21] The presence of both albumin and phospholipids in alveolar epithelial lining fluid may, therefore, be important constituents for facilitated epithelial cell uptake of nanoparticles after deposition in the alveolar space. After translocation to the blood circulation, nanoparticles can be distributed throughout the body.

3.1.3. Neural Uptake and Translocation

A translocation pathway for solid particles in the respiratory tract involves neuronal axons. The pathway for the nasal and tracheobronchial regions, comprise sensory nerve endings of the olfactory and the trigeminus nerves and an intricate network of sensory nerve endings in the tracheobronchial region. An inhalation study with nanosized manganese oxide (MnO_2) particles in rats showed a significant increase of Mn in the olfactory bulb[22]. However, bigger particles were unable to use the route since the individual axons of the olfactory nerve are only 100-200 nm in diameter[23,24]. Thus, olfactory nerve pathway should be considered a portal of entry to the CNS for humans. However, there are additional translocation pathways via the trigeminus nerve and tracheobronchial sensory nerves to the ganglion as shown by intranasally instilled particles.[25, 26]

3.2. Exposure via GI Tract and Skin

Nanoparticles cleared from the respiratory tract via the mucociliary escalator can subsequently be ingested into the GI tract. Alternatively, nanoparticles can be ingested directly if used as drugs or drug delivery devices. Most studies have shown that nanoparticles pass through the GI tract and are eliminated rapidly.[12,27] For example, in rats dosed orally with radiolabeled functionalized C_{60} fullerenes, water solubilized using PEG and albumin, 98% were cleared in the feces within 48 hrs, whereas the rest was eliminated via urine, indicating some uptake into the blood circulation.[27] Another potentially important uptake route is through dermal exposure. Studies in mice and pigs with intradermally injected near-infrared quantum dots for in vivo imaging confirmed that nanoparticles once in the dermis, will localize to regional lymph nodes likely with the help of skin macrophages and dendritic cells.[28] This raises a question about potential modulation of immune responses after interaction of these nanoparticle-containing macrophages and dendritic cells with T lymphocytes.[29]

3.3. Injection Route

Intravenous injection is a very useful way to deliver drugs. After intravenous delivery or by any other route, once the nanoparticles translocate to the blood circulation, the liver becomes the major distribution site via uptake by Kupifer cells, followed by the spleen as another organ of the reticuloendothelial system. However, coating with polyethylene glycol (PEG) almost completely prevents hepatic and splenic localization so that other organs can be targeted.[30] Distribution to the heart, kidney and immune-modulating organs (spleen, bone marrow) has been reported. For example, after intravenous injection in mice, 10 nm PEG-coated quantum dots appeared in liver, spleen, lymph nodes and bone marrow, <220 nm metallo-flullerene accumulated mainly in liver and bone marrow and 240 nm polystyrene (nonbiodegradable) and polylisohexylcyonacrylate (biodegradable) distributed in bone marrow and phagocytic cells.[31-35] Human serum albumin-coated polylactic acid nanoparticles (90-250 nm) were rapidly captured by liver, bone marrow, lymph nodes, spleen and peritoneal macrophages after parenteral administration to rat.[36] Targeting specificity is thus extremely valuable for drug delivery; thus, drug delivery to the CNS requires nanoparticle surface modification, for example, by coating with apolipoprotein for LDL-receptor-mediated endocytosis in brain capillaries.[37] So, desirable particle surface modification must be carefully weighted against potential adverse cellular responses of targeted drug delivery.

4. Biological Adverse Effects of Nanoparticles

The unique biokinetic behaviors of nanoparticles, such as cellular endocytosis, transcytosis, neuronal and circulatory translocation and distribution, which makes them desirable for medical therapeutic or diagnostic application, may be associated with potential toxicity. For example, nanoparticle-facilitated drug delivery to the CNS raises the question of the fate of nanoparticles after their translocation to specific cell types or to subcellular structures in the brain.

4.1. Pulmonary Effects of Nanoparticles

Due to either environmental exposure to nanoparticles, occupational production of nanoparticles or nasal delivery of nanoparticle-based drugs, the lung is a major target organ for particle-induced effects. For the interpretation of nanoparticle-mediated effects, five parameters have to be taken into account, i. e.: (1) Dose, (2) Deposition, (3) Dimension, (4) Durability and (5) Defense. First of all, the dose at a specific site in the lungs determines the potential toxicity. This deposited dose is dependent on the concentration and the dimensions of the particles. As mentioned before, the deposition probability of nanoparticles increases steeply in the respiratory tract as particle size decreases. If a particle is neither soluble nor degradable in the lung, it has a high durability and there will be rapid local accumulation upon sustained exposure. Although the lung has extensive defense systems such as mucociliary clearance (upper airways) and macrophage clearance (lower airways, alveoli) to remove deposited particles as described above, for nanoparticles, defense is not sufficient since their small size may prevent recognition by macrophages and sometimes surfaces are designed to behave as "stealth" particles, remaining unrecognized by phagocytosing cells.[38] Thus, nanoparticles can migrate to body compartments away from their application or deposited sites by other routes as explained before.

4.1.1. Pulmonary Inflammation

Among the mechanisms by which nanoparticles could cause an enhanced inflammatory response, direct effects have been reported on alveolar macrophages such as inward leaching of Ca^{2+}, impairment of phagocytosis and cytoskeletal changes.[39-41] Upon contact with nanoparticles, the cells in respiratory tract, such as macrophages, epithelial cells and neutrophilic granulocytes are activated to synthesize and secrete reactive oxygen species, cytokines and chemokines. Secreted cytokines and chemokines interact with specific receptors on the surface of many cell types and result in activation of local cells as well as those in the blood and other tissues. Thus, cells from the bloodstream are attracted to enter the fluid filled interstitial spaces, where they can attack the foreign material. Consequently, particle-induced cell activation events in the airways frequently result in an inflammatory response. A molecular mechanism for induction of inflammation has been shown in Fig. 1. Epithelial and nerve cells may also contribute to airway inflammation by producing pharmacologically active compounds, such as, capsacein.[42,43] In this neurogenic inflammation, stimulation of sensory nerve endings releases neurotransmitters which may affect many types of white blood cells in the lung, as well as epithelial and smooth muscle cells. Persistent or high inflammatory response may damage the epithelial cell layer at the surface of the tissue and other cells (such as macrophages), which can result in tissue damage and loss of function.

Thus, particle deposition on the respiratory epithelium can set off a cascade of events in many different cells, potentially resulting in diverse changes in tissues and organs at sites progressively further away from the initial stimulus. These changes are thought to have a greater impact on individuals whose respiratory, cardiac or vascular tissues have been previously compromised.

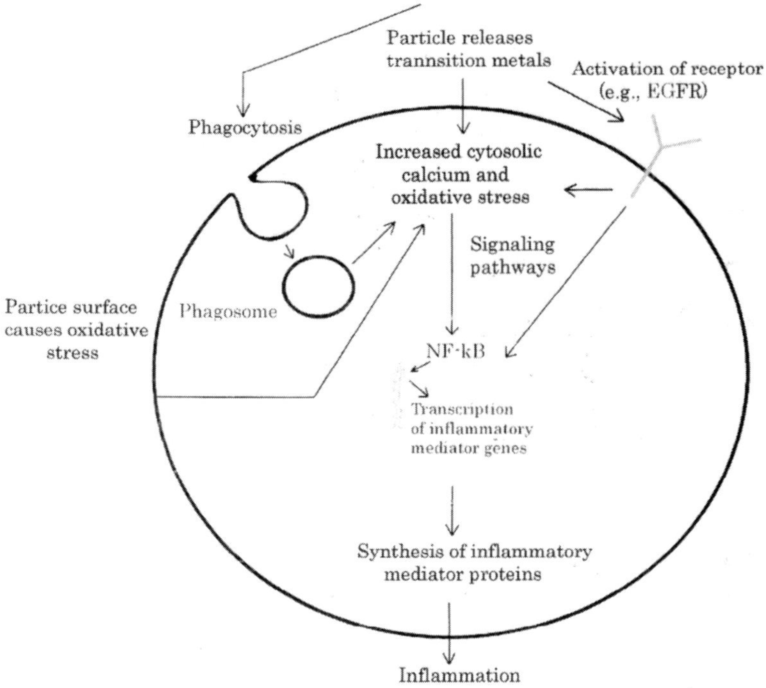

Figure 1. Molecular mechanism for the induction of inflammation.

4.1.2. Pulmonary Carcinogenicity

Low toxic poorly soluble particulates (PSP) such as carbon black and titanium dioxide (TiO_2) induce chronic inflammation, fibrosis, neoplastic lesions and lung tumors in rats.[44,45] Lung tumors associated with exposure to such particles are generally of two types, i. e., those originating from alveolar type II cells, called bronchoalveolar tumors and squamous or epidermoid tumors which are considered to arise with from areas of squamous metaplasia.[45] The tumors include adenomas (BA), adenocarcinomas (BAC), squamous cell carcinoma (SCC), adenosquamous carcinomas and squamous keratinizing cyst (SKC). The continued presence of high levels of non-toxic particle surface leads to the impairment of alveolar macrophage clearance, culminating in rapid buildup of particles, chronic inflammatory response, fibrosis and tumorigenesis. The inflammatory cell influx is responsible for the lung tumors after saturation of lung clearance by overloading of macrophages with PSP due to their mutagenic activity and actions on cell proliferation.[45, 47]

A schematic description of the stages thought to be involved in the pulmonary toxicity of poorly soluble particles is shown in Fig. 2.

4.2. Systemic Effects of Nanoparticles

Nanoparticles after reaching the blood circulation by any of the aforementioned routes, can be internalized in the cells throughout the body and, therefore, should be able to interact with signaling processes. Nanoparticles below 40 nm have a size similar to large proteins and so may form complexes with endogenous proteins and may complicate different endogenous proteins depending on nanoparticle surface properties. Different nanoparticle-protein complexes may have different biokinetics, including translocation across membranes and endogenous proteins of these complexes may have a different activity or even a different function.[48] If the particle is not degradable and its size is above 5 nm, the particle can not be cleared through renal elimination and so may exert more adverse effects in the body. Among the indirect effects, inflammation in the lung due to particle deposition may affect target organs by mediators that become systemically available. The inflammatory mediators may trigger systemic hypercoagulability of the blood, thereby increasing the risk for cardiovascular events.[49] Progression of atherosclerosis and increased vulnerability to plaque rupture has also been suggested for particle inhalation-mediated cardiovascular death.[50] Nanoparticles may also affect CNS since they can be transported along axial nerve endings to the brain (mentioned above).

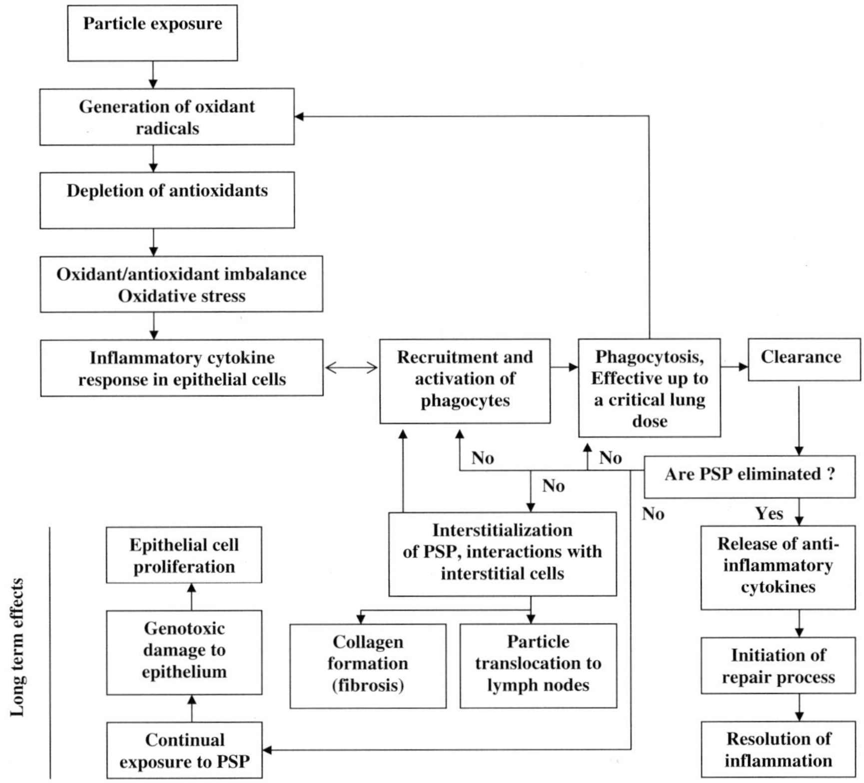

Figure 2. Schematic description of the stages thought to be involved in the pulmonary toxicity of poorly soluble particles.

4.3. Differences in Toxicity between Nanoparticles of Different Materials

The toxicity of inhaled poorly soluble particles has been clearly established with smaller particles eliciting a greater pulmonary inflammatory response than do larger particles on a mass basis for the same material. However, two other factors have been proposed to be involved in determining the respiratory tract response to particle exposure.

4.3.1. Particle Surface Activity

This is specifically the ability of the particle surface to generate free radicals.[51] When metallic cobalt (20 nm), metallic nickel (20 nm) and TiO_2 (28 nm) nanoparticles of similar specific surface areas were instilled in equal mass doses in a rat, nickel demonstrated significantly greater inflammatory responses than either cobalt or TiO_2 and cobalt was more inflammogenic than TiO_2.[52] Nickel also produced a marked increase in lymphocytes in bronchoalveolar lavage fluid (BALF). Nickel and cobalt but not TiO_2 caused lipid peroxidation. With respect to free radical generating ability in vitro, TiO_2 showed little free radical producing activity while nickel and cobalt showed similar free (hydroxyl) radical production activity. Thus, free radical generating potential may be one element that determines inflammatory potential and pulmonary toxicity.

4.3.2. Particle Agglomeration/Disagglomeration

This is a determinant of the availability of individual particles to the lung surface once the material has entered the lung.[53] Particles tend to agglomerate and the extent to which disagglomeration occurs once particles enter the lung may influence the subsequent toxicity since the routes of particle translocation from the site of deposition is dependent on particle diameter as described before.

5. Conclusions

The introduction of nanostructured materials opens tremendous opportunities for biomedical applications as therapeutic and diagnostic tools. However, very little is known about their potential to cause adverse effects or humoral immune responses once they are introduced into the organism either unintentionally or intentionally. The lack of toxicology data on engineered nanoparticles does not allow for adequate risk assessment. Rigorous assessment of biocompatibility according to the guidelines provided by the regulatory agencies is, therefore, necessary to identify potential hazards in order to develop a scientifically defensible database for the purpose of risk assessment. Sufficient resources should be allocated by governmental agencies and industries to be able to perform a scientifically based risk assessment and then establish justifiable procedures for risk management.

Bibliography

1. Delarnothe T. (2005) Nanotechnology: small science, big deal. *British Medical Journal* **330**: 544.
2. Biological Evaluation of Medical Devices, ISO 10993 Standard Series, Geneva, International Organization for Standardization, ongoing.
3. Bollen L S and Svendsen O. (1997). Regulatory guidelines for biocompatibility safety testing. *Medical Plastic and Biomaterials.*
4. Anderson J M. (2001) Biological responses to materials. *Annu Rev Mater Res* **31**: 81-110.
5. Oberdorster C, Oberdorster E, and Oberdorster J. (2005) Nanotoxicology: an emerging discipline evolving from studies of ultrafine particles. *Environmental Health Perspectives* **113**: 823-839.
6. Oberdorster G. (2005) Principles for characterizing the potential human health effects from exposure to nanomaterials: elements of a screening strategy. *Particle and Fibre Toxicology* **2**(**1-3**): 5.
7. Kreyling W G and Scheuch G (2000) Clearance of particles deposited in the lungs. In: *Particle-Lung Interactions* Gehr P and Heyder J (eds.) Marcel Dekker Inc., New York, NY 323-376, 2000.
8. Schlesinger R B. (1997) Disposition of inhaled toxicants. In: *Handbook of Human Toxicology* Massaro EJ (ed). CRC Press, New York, NY 493-550.
9. Warheit D B, Overby L H, George G and Brody A R. (1988) Pulmonary macrophages are attracted to inhaled particles on alveolar surfaces. *Exp. Lung Res* **14**: 51-66.
10. Warheit D B, Hill L H, George O and Brody A R. (1986) Time course of chemotactic factor generation and the corresponding macrophage response to asbestos inhalation. *Am Rev Respir Dis* **134**: 128-133.
11. Warheit D B and Hartsky M A. (1993) Role of alveolar macrophage chemotaxis and phagocytosis in pulmonary clearance responses to inhaled particles: comparisons among rodent species. *Microsc Res Tech* **26**: 412-422.
12. Kreyling W. (2002) Translocation of ultrafine insoluble iridium particles from lung epithelium to extrapulmonary organs is size dependent but very low. *J Toxicol Environ Health* **65**: 1513-153.
13. Oberdorster G. (2000) Toxicology of ultrafine particles: in vivo studies. *Philos Trans R Soc Lond A* **358**: 2719-2740.

14. Semmler M. (2004) Long-term clearance kinetics of inhaled ultrafine insoluble iridium particles from the rat lung, including transient translocation into secondary organs. *Inhal Toxicol* **16**: 453-459.
15. Oberdorster O. (1992) Role of the alveolar macrophage in lung injury: studies with ultrafine particles. *Environ Health Perspect* **97**: 193-197.
16. Ferin J and Oberdorster G. (1992) Translocation of particles from pulmonary alveoli into the interstitium. *J. Aerosol Med* **5**: 179-187.
17. Nikula K I, Avila KI, Griffith W C, Mauderly I L. (1997) Lung tissue responses and sites of particle retention differ between rats and cynomolgus monkeys exposed chronically to diesel exhaust and coal dust. *Fundam Appl Toxicol* **37**: 37-53.
18. Berry J P, Arnoux B, Stanislas O, Galle P and Chretien J A. (1997) Microanalytical study particles transport across the alveoli: role of blood platelets. *Biomedicine* **27**: 354-357.
19. Mehta D, Bhattacharya I, Matthay M A and Malik A B. (2004) Integrated control of lung fluid balance. *Am Physiol Lung Cell Mol Physiol* **287**: L1081-L1090.
20. Heckel K, Kiefmann R, Dorger M, Stoeckeihuber M. and Goetz A E. (2004) Colloidal gold particles as a new in vivo marker of early acute lung injury. *Am J Physiol Lung Cell Mol Physiol* **287**: L867-L878.
21. Kato T. (2003) Evidence that exogenous substances can be phagocytosed by alveolarepithelial cells and transported into blood capillaries. *Cell Tiss Res* **311**: 47-51.
22. Feikert T. (2004) Inhaled solid ultrafine particles (UFP) are efficiently translocated via neuronal naso-olfactory pathways. *Toxicologist* **78 (suppl 1)**: 43 5-436.
23. Fechter L D, Johnson D L and Lynch R A. (2002) The relationship of particle size to olfactory nerve uptake of a non-soluble form of magnesium into brain. *Neurotoxicology* **23**: 177-183.
24. Plattig KH. (1989) Electrophysiology of taste and smell. *Clin Phys Physiol Meas* **10**: 91-126.
25. Hunter D D. and Dey R D. (1998) Identification and neuropeptide content of trigeminal neurons innervating the rat nasal epithelium. *Neuroscience* **83**: 591-599.
26. Hunter D D and Undem B J. (1943-1948) Identification and substance P contentofvagal afferent neurons innervating the epithelium of the guinea pig trachea. *Am J Respir Crit Care Med* **159**.
27. Yamago S. (1995) In vivo biological behavior of a water-miscible fullerene: labeling, absorption, distribution, excretion and acute toxicity. *Chem Biol* **2**: 385-389.
28. Oh L. (2004) CCR7 governs skin dendritic cell migration under inflammatory and steady-state conditions. *Immunity* **21**: 279-288.
29. Chen B, Wilson S, Das M, Coughlin D and Erlanger B. (2000) Antigenicity of fullerenes: antibodies specific for flullerenes and their characteristics. *Proc Nat Acad Sci USA* **95**: 10809-10813.

30. Akerman M A, Chan W C W, Laakkonen P, Bhatia S N and Ruoslahti E. (2002) Nanocrystal targeting in vivo. *Proc Natl Acad Sd USA* **99**: 12617-12621.
31. Ballou B, Lagerhoim B C, Ernst L A, Bruchez M P, Waggoner A S. (2004) Non-invasive imaging of quantum dots in mice. *Bioconjugate Chem* **15**: 79-86.
32. Cagle D W, Kenmnel S J, Mirzadeh S, Alford J M and Wilson L J. (1999) In vivo studies of fullerene-based materials using endohedral metallofullerene radiotracers. *Proc Nat Acad Sci USA* **96**: 5 182-5187.
33. Gibaud S. (1996) Cells involved in the capture of nanoparticles in hematopoietic organs. *J Pharm Sci* **85**: 944-950.
34. Gibaud S. (1998) Polyalkylcyanoacrylate nanoparticles as carriers for granulocyte-colony stimulating (G-CSF). *J. Control. Release* **52**: 131-139.
35. Gibaud S. (1994) Increased bone marrow toxicity of doxorubicin bound to nanoparticles. *Eur. J. Cancer* **30A**: 820-826.
36. Bazile D V. (1992) Body distribution of filly biodegradable [14C]-poly(lactic acid) nanoparticles coated with albumin after parenteral administration to rats. *Biomaterials* 13: 1093-1102.
37. Kreuter J. (2002) Apolipoprotein-mediated transport of nanoparticle-bound drugs across the blood-brain barrier. *J Drug Target* **10**: 3 17-325.
38. Moghimi S M and Hunter A C. (2001) Capture of stealth nanoparticles by the body's defenses. *Crit Reb Ther Drug Camer Syst* **18**: 527.
39. Stone V. (2000) Increased calcium influx in a monocytic cell line on exposure to ultrafine carbon black. *Eur Respir Journal* **15**: 297-303.
40. Renwick L C, Donaldson K and Clouter A. (2001) Impairment of alveolar macrophage phagocytosis by ultrafine particles. *Toxicol Appl Pharmacol* **172**: 119-127.
41. Molter W, Hofer T, Ziesenis A, Karg E and Heyder J. (2002) Ultrafine particles cause cytoskeletal dysfunctions in macrophages. *Toxicolology and Applied Pharmacology* **182**: 197-207.
42. Barnes P J. (2001) Neurogenic inflammation in the airways. *Respir Physiol* **125**: 145-154.
43. Veronesi B, de Haar C, Roy J and Oortgiesen M. (2002) Particulate matterinflammation and receptor sensitivity are target cell specific. *Inhal Toxico* **14**: 159-183.
44. Nikula K J. (2000) Rat lung tumors induced by exposure to selected poorly soluble nonfibrous particles. *Inhal Toxicol* **12**: 97-119.
45. Greim H. (2001) Toxicity of fibers and particles. Report of the workshop held in Munich, Germany, 26-27 October 2000. *Inhal Toxicol* **13**: 737-754.
46. Hext P M. (1994) Current perspectives on particulate induced pulmonary tumours. *Human Exp Toxicol* **13**: 700-715.
47. Driscoll K E. (1997) Effects of particle exposure and particle-elicited inflammatory cells on mutation in rat alveolar epithelial cells. *Carcinogenesis* **18**: 423-430.

48. Borm P J A and Kreyling W. (2004) Toxicology hazards of inhaled nanoparticles-Potential implications for drug delivery. *Journal of Nanoscience and Nanotechnology* **4**: 1-11.
49. Seaton A and MacNee W, Donaldson K and Godden D. (1995) Particulate air pollution and acute health effects. *Lancet* **345**: 176-178.
50. Suwa T. (2005) Particulate air pollution induces progression of atherosclerosis. *Journal of Nanoscience and Nanotechnology* **4**: 12-21.

Chapter 8

Nanoparticles: Effects on Human Health and the Environment

Myung-Haing Cho and Jin-Kyu Lee

1. Hopes and Concerns about Nanotechnology

Nanomaterials are defined as materials that have at least one dimension in the 1 to 100 nm range. Nano-sized materials can be produced naturally during forest fires and volcanic activity and can exist as viral particles, biogenic magnetite, and even as biomolecules such as ferritin.[1] Numerous man-made nano-sized materials exist unintentionally as produced from combustion by-products or intentionally as produced as manufactured nanomaterials. Among such diverse sources of nanomaterials, manufactured nanomaterials are under scrutiny for their applications in diverse areas such as electronic and photonic devices, medicine, drug delivery system, and diagnostic imaging applications. In this chapter, the potential concerns of manufactured nanomaterials are emphasized because other sources of nanomaterials are not produced intentionally. Manufactured nanomaterials are used in diverse applications and, thus, are exposed to diverse human and environmental conditions. The rapid development in nanotechnology will result in several changes in the areas such as nanoscale visualization, insights into how living systems operate, revolutionary biotechnology, synthesis of new drugs in targeted delivery applications, and regenerative medicine; all offer many benefits.[1]

The recent shift in the focus of developing materials from microscale to nanoscale is essential for future advances in both digital and biological applications and may change the foundations of education, medicine, and industrial manufacturing, while having potential harmful effects on the environment. Reducing particle size of materials is an efficient and reliable tool for improving the bioavailability of a gene or drug delivery system. In fact, nanotechnology helps in overcoming the pre-existing limitations of size.[1] The surface of nanomaterials can be further modified to improve their efficiency and facilitate their applications in many important different fields of bioscience and medicine. Much effort is being devoted to the creation of new materials on the nanometer scale in the hopes of improving clinical diagnosis and therapy. In order to prevent potential adversities, however, it is necessary to collect more information on the toxicological consequences of nanomaterials and to investigate any possible side effects of these nanomaterials before introducing such materials into humans. This is important since several examples of current nanomaterials contain toxic elements which may be release toxic ions upon corrosion. These nanomaterials may show unexpected new biological activities as a result of their small size (having an activated surface). Generally, nanomaterials are ingested in a nonspecific way by cells, and thus, by living organisms.

Nanotechnologies contain almost unlimited potentials for improving medical applications, such as in cancer biology. Cancer-related examples of nanotechnologies include injectable drug-delivery nanovectors, such as liposomes for the therapy of breast cancer; biologically targeted and nanosized magnetic nanoparticles for drug delivery as well as molecular imaging; and novel and biocompatible nanoparticle-based aerosol gene delivery for lung cancer treatment.[2-4] In an ideal scheme, the onset of the transformational processes leading towards malignancy should be detected early, as a matter of routine screening, by noninvasive means such as proteomic analysis from blood, or by *in vivo* imaging of molecular profiles and evolving lesion configurates. The detailed biology of the host and the disease should be accurately elucidated, and dictate choices for targeting and barrier-avoiding revolutionary strategies for an intervention plan. Transforming cellular populations should be reduced or prevented without collateral effects on healthy cells and tissues. Cancer treatment efficacy should be monitored in real time to assess therapeutic effects *in situ*. If fully integrated with established cancer-research activities, nanotechnology may help this innovative vision become reality. Developing approaches for the *in vivo* detection and monitoring of cancer biomarkers, refining technology for early detection of cancer biomarkers, improving the targeting efficacy of therapeutic or imaging agents to cancer lesions and their microenvironment can be exploited with engineered nanomaterials. These materials can avoid biological and biophysical barriers, and regulatory issues, thus, provide promising opportunities for the application of nanotechnology. Taken together, nanotechnology in combination with modern science may synergistically play important roles in realizing the goals of detecting and treatment of transforming cell populations early *in vivo* or *ex vivo*. Nanomaterials will also provide information regarding appropriate combinations of agents and particle specific targeting of these agents to early cancer lesions to eliminate or suppress them without adverse effects on healthy tissues. Nanoparticles could provide useful real-time information for staging, and monitoring treatment effects.

Living systems utilize regulatory systems that are governed at the nanometer scale. Recent insights into the uses of nanofabricated devices and systems (such as protein-chip and lab-on-a-chip) with self-assembly systems strongly suggest that processes of genome sequence and detection of gene expression can be made efficiently through the use of nanofabricated materials and devices. Moreover, in addition to facilitating optimal drug usage, nanotechnology can provide new formulations and efficient routes for drug delivery, thus, providing additional layers of drug concentration and control at the molecular level, thereby improving accuracy in treatment and broadening the therapeutical efficacy of drugs of interest.

Such an increasing nanotechnological revolution will also definitely benefit all basic studies of cell biology and pathology. As a result of the development of new analytical tools capable of probing the world of nanometer beyond normal scale, it will be clearly possible to characterize the chemical and physico-mechanical properties of cells and organisms and to measure mechanistic and dynamic properties of single molecules. With these dramatic developments, nanotechnologies should complement the ensemble all traditional common techniques presently used in the modern biology and life sciences. Moreover, such developed nanotechnology-derived highly controllable nanostructures can produce biocompatible, high-performance materials with tremendous application in areas such as single cell manipulation, specific targeting/curing, and high throughput screening (HTS). Artificial inorganic and organic nanoscale materials can be also introduced into cells or organs to play key roles in molecular diagnostics and therapeutics. Finally, nanotechnology-enabled Information Technology (IT)-Biotechnology (BT) fusion will increase computational power, thus, permit the characterization of macromolecular networks in a realistic environment. Such fusion technology-based simulations will be essential for developing biocompatible materials applicable to living organisms and for studying new drug discovery processes. An un-defined and critical issue is how nanoparticles will affect health and the environment and how we can predict and prevent illness, or damage, prior to exposure.

As mentioned above, nanoscience and nanotechnology have high potential to bring invaluable benefits in diverse areas. They are attracting rapidly increasing investments from government and industry in many parts of world. Simultaneously though, such rapid and widespread applications of nanomaterials may confer substantial potential concerns for human exposure and environmental release. Therefore, the future of nanotechnology may depend upon public acceptance of the risk versus benefits as has been observed with genetically modified organisms. In fact, the key issues are the appropriate basis of evaluating and regulating nanomaterials in order to protect humans and the environment.

2. Possible Adverse Health, Environment, and Safety Impacts

To understand the potential adverse effects of nanomaterials on health, one must understand the general defense mechanism of living organisms and the interactions between these particles and the immune responses. Based on much of evolutionary history, humans have been exposed to small particles and, thus, have developed defense mechanisms against such particles. As shown in Fig. 1, dominant routes of access to humans are organs such as the lung (inhalation), skin (contact) or intestine (swallowing) which contain barriers to penetration by small particles. Regardless of the presence of such defense mechanisms, nanosized materials may present problems for humans because defense mechanisms may not work properly against nanosize materials. Mineral quartz, asbestos and particles associated with air pollution are the representative examples of such nanomaterials.

Medical applications of nanoparticles can be another source of adversity on human health. For many years scientists have studied the biological fate of nanoscale particles with the aim of developing novel drug delivery systems. Several lines of recent evidences imply that some nanoscale materials may penetrate into cells, thus, toxicity tests need to take into account these potential interactions of medical nanomaterials such as cosmetics including sunscreens. Although there is some limited evidence about the human impacts of nanoparticles, research on the impacts of nanomaterials on the natural environment and on non-human species is not sufficient.

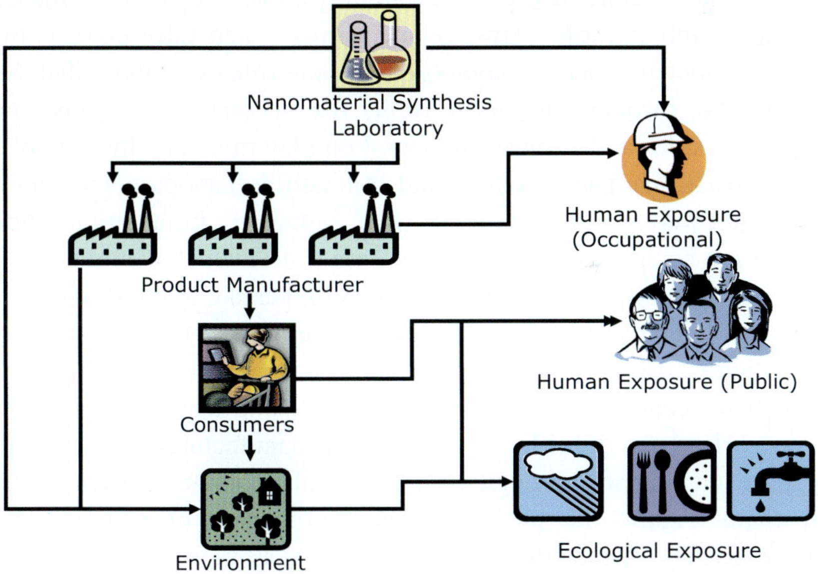

Figure 1. Potential routes of exposure to nanomaterials to humans and the environment.

Recently, comparative studies have been performed to test the potential differences in toxicity from inhaled versus intraperitoneal exposures to magnetic nanoparticles. This study indicates that intraperitoneal administration of 50 nm silica-coated magnetic nanoparticles did not cause apparent toxicity, however, inhalation administration did. Most likely, first-pass effects by the portal circulation would reduce toxicities from intra-peritoneal routes, however, detailed information for the differential toxicity remains unknown.[4] Furthermore, there is only one published study of the impact of manufactured nanoparticles on non-human species other than laboratory animals. In this study, a significant increase of lipid peroxidation was found in the brain of juvenile largemouth bass exposed to 0.5 ppm C_{60} fullerene nanoparticles.[6]

Although beyond the scope of this chapter, it is important to keep in mind the potential role of atmospheric nanoparticles in photocatalytic and thermal production of atmospheric pollutants. Atmospheric aerosols in heavily polluted areas have the potential to accelerate ozone formation reactions. Furthermore, because they are respirable, they could represent a serious health hazard. Atmospheric aerosols generally contain two major components: one is composed of amorphous carbon that has fullerene-like particles dispersed in it; the second is inorganic and consists of oxides and sulfides supported on clay minerals. In particular, the iron oxide, manganese oxide, and iron sulfide nanoparticles tend to have photocatalytic adsorption of solar radiation. In addition, these materials are acidic and may be coated with water, which would enhance their catalytic ability to crack hydrocarbons and create free radicals.[7] It is also plausible that soil or water organisms can uptake the manufactured nanoparticles escaping into the natural environment and such nanoparticles can disturb vital functions depending upon characteristics such as surface activity. Moreover, released manufactured nanoparticles may re-reach humans through environmental ecosystems such as the food chain. Again, the physicochemical properties of nanomaterials would determine the environmental fate such as bioaccumulation and persistence.

3. How to Evaluate the Toxicity of Nanoparticles?

As mentioned earlier, nanomaterials are expected to improve virtually all areas of science and commercializing products. However, such widespread application of nanomaterials may cause significant potentials for human exposure and environmental release. Therefore, appropriate risk assessment and management of nanomaterials should be performed to assess and regulate these nanomaterials to protect human health and the environment (Figure 2). While ingestion and skin penetration are potential exposure routes for engineered nanomaterials, the inhalation route has perhaps received the most attention.[1] In this section, general aspects for appropriate toxicity evaluation of nanomaterials will be evaluated.

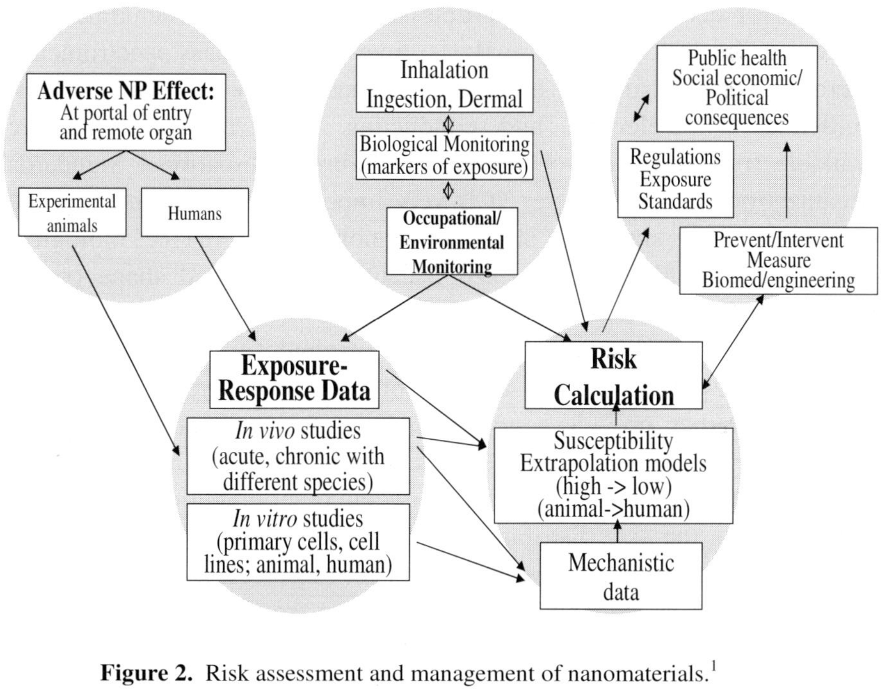

Figure 2. Risk assessment and management of nanomaterials.[1]

First of all, characterization of nanomaterials is essential because the reactivity of surface atoms depends highly upon the size, shape and morphology, and adsorbed chemical. Complete characterization of nanoparticles includes such measurements as size, size distribution, shape and other morphological features, chemistry of the materials, solubility, surface area, state of dispersion, surface chemistry and other physicochemical properties. Exhaustive characterization of test nanomaterials may be time consuming, expensive and complex. Therefore, an agreeable basis of minimum characteristics should be included for the safety evaluation of nanomaterials. Such a basis includes size, shape, state of dispersion, physical and chemical properties, surface area, and surface chemistry.[8]

As mentioned earlier, the definition of a nanomaterial has been generally agreed upon to include any material with at least one dimension smaller than 100 nanometers. Therefore, reliable methods for size measurements should be developed. There are a wide variety of methods for determining nanoparticle size distributions, including light scattering, dynamic mobility analysis, time-of-flight mass spectrometry, microscopy, and surface area measurements, among many others. Guidelines for selecting and conducting these measurements are available from a variety of sources, including International Standards Organization (ISO). However, it is very important to recognize that the measurement of size and shape of nanomaterials in the biological environment should be performed because the size and shape of the nanomaterial interacting with a biomolecule in living organism or with others may differ dramatically from its original form. For example, nanoparticles produced from an aerosol particle generator for animal inhalation studies provide a good prototype. Upon creation through a generator, nanoparticles may begin to agglomerate according to their size, concentration, temperature, pressure and other conditions.

Therefore, the size distribution "as exposed" or "as dosed" may be quite different from that of "as generated" or "as received." How can we avoid such unexpected changes? In fact, there are no definitive answers to the question. The best available methods are to carefully consider the potential implications of the administration methods, attempt to be realistic in terms of exposure conditions and make the best measurements possible. Assessing the degree of dispersion in the biological environment is a function of the ability to make size distribution measurements. Size distribution measurements are feasible in simulated biological fluids, however, there are few techniques available to directly measure agglomerated size in living cells or tissues. Post-mortem microscopy is one of the basic techniques for qualitatively assessing the state of dispersion. For example, Fig. 3 shows a TEM micrograph of silica-coated magnetic nanoparticles ($MNP@SiO_2$) inside a lung cancer cell. Individual particles and agglomerates are evident, however, it remains unclear whether agglomeration takes place before or after the particles are taken up by cells.

Physical and chemical properties of nanomaterials include a wide range of particle characteristics such as elemental composition, chemical reactivity, solubility, and physico-chemical constants. For many nanomaterials, such properties seem to be same as those of conventional scale material. However, it is also possible that the physicochemical properties of nanomaterials may be changed as the particle size decreases. Thus, one should consider the toxicity of nanomaterials even though the original material at the conventional scale is not toxic. Especially, such properties of nanomaterials in biological fluid should not be ignored. Physicochemical properties of nanomaterials are known to be a function of the particle itself and its environment. Thus, characteristics of particles should be measured under the conditions of biological fluids such as *ex vivo* physiological fluids or *in vitro* solutions.

Interactions between nanomaterials and biological organisms typically take place at the surface of nanomaterials, thus, surface area seems to be one of the primary factors in determining toxicity. Surface area can be characterized in 2 ways; external surface area and internal surface area (porosity). The external and internal surface areas of nanomaterials can be measured by gas adsorption methods, surface titrations and aerosol diffusion.[9,10] It is important to know that the practical surface area and porosity of nanomaterials in biological environment can be changed due to potential adsorption of biomolecules or self-agglomeration. Such changes may affect the toxicity of nanomaterials. Surface charge of nanomaterials is also critical to determine the toxicity because it is a major factor in determining the particle dispersion characteristics and will influence the adsorption and interaction with biomolecules in living organism.

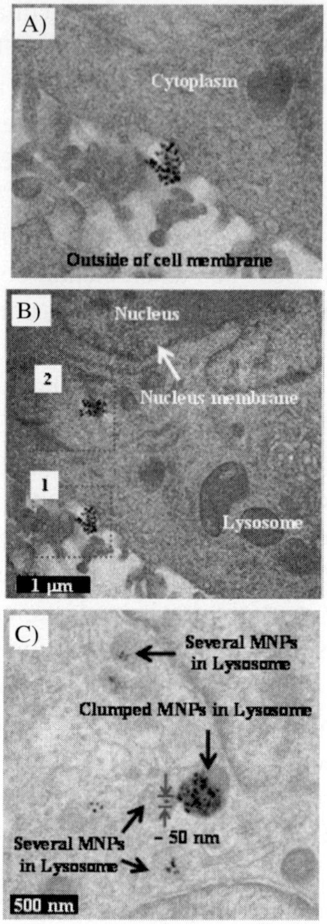

Figure 3. Representative transmission electron micrographs (TEM) of A549 cells treated with silica-coated magnetic nanoparticles**.** To elucidate the detailed information of MNP@SiO_2 uptake through endocome-lysosomal mechanism, a TEM study was performed. The treated cells were fixed with glutaraldehyde, paraformaldehyde, and osmium tetroxide and embedded with epoxy resin. Thin sections were made using ultramicrotome and not stained with any reagent for detecting the uptake of nanoparticles into the cells. Images were collected using a transmission electron microscope and digital camera. (A) Uptake of silica-coated MNPs was initiated by starting the invagination of the plasma membrane. (B) Some nanoparticles were already internalized into the cells (solid line box 2) while the cells still are uptaking at the plasma membrane (solid line box 1). (C) Uptaken silica-coated magnetic nanoparticles were trapped inside the lysosome.

4. Conclusions

Many applications of nanotechnologies should not produce adverse effects on human health and the environment. To predict and prevent the potential toxicity of nanomaterials, therefore, the complete characterization of nanomaterials should be measured under conditions as close to the point of application as possible. For toxicity studies, this should include the biological environment. For example, the particle size should be measured in cell culture media or at least under the same pH and ionic strength conditions as observed *in vivo*. Exposure to natural or man-made nanomaterials in ambient conditions and indoor could be unavoidable, and most of the population and workers in many industries seem to be exposed to nanomaterials. There is no clear and direct evidence that such exposure may be responsible for the observed relationships between air pollution and several diseases in susceptible individuals. Objectively, it seems likely that the needs of industry will be met by development of various nanomaterials with different physico-chemical properties. Therefore, new manufactured nanomaterials should be treated with caution and evaluated for toxic potential.

Until research has been undertaken to establish the appropriate battery of toxicity tests, it may not be possible to evaluate the potential impacts on humans and the environment. Until more is known about such impacts, it is highly recommended that the manufacture and release of nanomaterials should be regulated through multifunctional activities among academia, governmental regulatory agencies and industries as shown in the following Fig. 4. Our suggestion is based on incomplete information about the toxicology and epidemiology of manufactured nanomaterials and their behavior in environment. Therefore, it is highly recommended that extensive and multidisciplinary collaborative research of the impacts of nanomaterials into human and environment should keep pace with the predicted development. Therefore, we recommend that interdisciplinary research centers, composed of highly qualified research personnel, should be established in order to undertake research into the toxicity, epidemiology, efficacy, and environmental impacts and in order to communicate closely with governmental regulatory agencies.

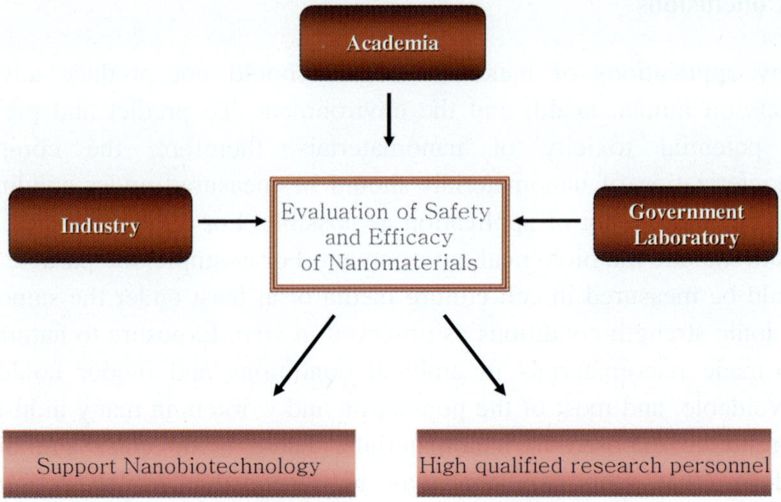

Figure 4. Schematic diagram of the establishment of interdisciplinary research centers for safety assurance of anomaterials

Acknowledgements

Part of preparing current chapter is supported by Nano Systems Institute-National Core Research Center (NSI-NCRC) in Korea. Authors would like to express our deep thanks to Dr. Jeff Lakritz of Ohio State University for his careful review of current chapter.

Bibliography

1. Oberdorster G, Oberdorster E, Oberdorster J. (2005) Nanotoxicology: an emerging discipline from studies of ultrafine particles. *Environ Health Perspect* 113: 823-839.
2. Park JW. (2002) Liposome-based drug delivery in breast cancer treatment. *Breast Cancer Res* **4**: 95-99.
3. Yoon TJ, Kim JS, Kim BG, Yu KN, Cho MH, Lee JK. (2005) Multifunctional magnetic nanoparticles possessing "magnetic motor effect" for drug or gene delivery. *Angew Chem Int Ed Engl* **44(7)**: 1068-1071.
4. Kim JS, Yoon TJ, Yu KN, Kim BG, Park SJ, Kim HW, Lee KH, Park SB, Lee JK, Cho MH. (2006) Toxicity and tissue distribution of magnetic nanoparticles in mice. *Tox Sci* **89(1)**: 338-347.

5. Guo P. (2005) RNA nanotechnology: engineering, assembly and applications in detection, gene delivery and therapy. *J Nanosci Nanotechnol* **5(12)**: 1964-1982.
6. Oberdorster E. (2004) Manufactured nanomaterials (fullerenes, C60) induce oxidative stress in the brain of juvenile largemouth bass. *Environ Health Perspect* **112**: 1058-1062.
7. Chianelli RR. (1998) Synthesis, fundamental properties and applications of nanocrystals, sheets, and fullerenes based on layered transition metal chalcogenides. In *R&D Status and Trends*, (Siegel E., ed), Wiley, Hooboken, NJ.
8. Powers KW, Brown SC, Krishna VB, Wasdo SC, Moudgil BM, Roberts SM. (2007) Research strategies for safety evaluation of nanomaterials, Part 6: Characterization of nanoscale particles for toxicological evaluation. *Toxicol Sci* in press.
9. Allen T. (2004) Particle size measurement. *Vol. II: Surface Area and Pore Size Determination* 5th *Ed.* Chapman&Hall, New York, NY.
10. Burtscher H (2005) Physical characterization of particulate emissions from diesel engines: a review. *J Aerosol Sci* **36**: 896-932.
11. Ferrari M. (2005) Cancer Nanotechnology: Opportunities and Challeneges. *Nat Rev Cancer* **5(3)**: 161-171.
12. Kim HW, Park IK, Cho CS, Lee KH, Beck GRJr, Colburn NH, Cho MH. (2004) Aerosol gene delivery of glucosylated polyethyleneimine/phosphatase and tensin homologue deleted on chromosome 10 complex suppressed Akt downstream pathways in the lungs of K-ras null mice. *Cancer Res* **64(21)**: 7971-7976.

Index

acute systemic toxicity 203
allografts 12
alveolar macrophage-mediated clearance 208
Alzheimer's diseases 143
anisotropic bone 3
anodization 81
anodization processing parameters 82
arterial system 181
arterial wall 182
astrocytes 140
atherosclerosis 185
autografts 12
axons 140

balloon angioplasty 187
bioactive ceramics 25
biocompatibility for bone 15
biocompatibility testing 202
biodegradability for bone 16
biological properties of anodized metals 97
blood brain barrier 137
blood cells 185
bone cytokines 5
bone growth factors 5
bone impurities 6
bone modeling unit 8
bone sialoprotein 5
bone structure 3
brain 136

cancellous bone 3
carbon nanotubes composites 118
carbon nanotubes/nanofibers for bone 64, 116
carcinogenicity 205
cell recognition of implant surfaces 57
ceramics for bone 19
chemical composition through anodization 92
cochlear implant 162
collagen 3
composites for bone 19
computer brain interface 164
corrosion resistance 96
cortical bone 3
cytotoxicity 202

developmental toxicity 206
drug delivery
- conventional 153
- nanotechnology 155

electronic tissue interface 161
emulsion freeze drying 36
endothelial cells 183
environmental affects 224
epithelial entry of nanoparticles 208

fiber meshes and fiber bonding 39
fibroblasts 184
fibronectin 114

functional electrical stimulation 165
functionalized nanomaterials 70

gas foaming particulate leaching 33
genotoxicity 204
GI tract exposure 210
glia 139

Haversian systems 3
health affects 224
helical rosette nanotubes 63
hemacompatibility 205
hydroxyapatite 6

immune response 206
influence of chemistry on bone growth 57
influence of topography on bone growth 60
injection of nanoparticles 210
insulin-like growth factors 5
intracutaneous reactivity 203
iron oxide nanoparticles 155
irritation 203

lamellae 3

mechanical properties of bone 7
mechanical properties of metals 13
mechanical properties of polymers 24
melt molding 39
memory cognitive functions 166
metal alloys in bone 12
metals in bone 12
micron roughness through anodization 83
micropatterning of carbon nanotubes 126
multiple sclerosis 146, 151

nanocomposites 2
nanomaterial nanoroughness 118
nanomaterial surface energy 119
nanomaterial surface roughness 68
nanomaterial wettability 67
nanoparticle exposure 225
nanoroughness through anodization 85
nanostructured vascular 191
nanostructured vascular stents 190
nanotechnology and stem cells 156
nanotechnology treatments for the nervous system 148
nervous system anatomy 135
neural uptake of nanoparticles 209
neurological disorders 141
neurons 139

oscillating field stimulator 166
osteoblast differentiation 10
osteoblasts 9, 115
osteoclasts11
osteocytes 11
osteogenesis imperfecta 1
osteoinductivity 17
osteomalacia 1
osteon 3
osteonectin 5
osteopontin 5
osteoporosis 1
oxidized titanium 79

Paget's disease 1
particle agglomeration 216
PCL 24
PLGA degradation 22
PLGA for bone 19
polymers for bone 19
PPF 24
problems with current bone implants 55
procollagen 4
protein adsorption 111
protein properties 113

pulmonary carcinogenicity 213
pulmonary effects of nanoparticles 211
pulmonary inflammation 212

quantum dots 160

rapid prototyping 40
rationale for nanocomposites for bone 27
reproductive toxicity 206
respiratory entry of nanoparticles 207
rickets 1
risk assessment of nanoparticles 227

safety assurance of nanomaterials 232
sensitization 203
skeletal complications 54
skin exposure to nanoparticles 210
smooth muscle cells 184
solvent-casting particulate leaching 30
spinal cord 136
spinal cord injury 141
stem cell differentiation 116
stem cells 156
stent wear debris 193
stents 187
stress shielding 13
subchronic and chronic toxicity 205
superparamagnetic iron oxide nanoparticles 159
surface properties for bone 16
systemic effects of nanoparticles 214

tartrate resistant acid phosphatase 11
tissue engineering bone 13
tissue engineering fabrication techniques 18
toxicity 201
type I collagen 4

vascular stents 187
vascular system 181
visual prosthesis 163

woven bone 6

xenografts 12